CLINICAL SKILLS
FOR NURSES

Student Survival Skills Series

Survive your nursing course with these essential guides for all student nurses:

Calculation Skills for Nurses
Claire Boyd
9781118448892

Medicine Management Skills for Nurses
Claire Boyd
9781118448854

Clinical Skills for Nurses
Claire Boyd
9781118448779

CLINICAL SKILLS
FOR NURSES

Claire Boyd
RGN, Cert Ed
Practice Development Trainer

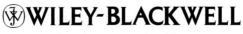

A John Wiley & Sons, Ltd., Publication

This edition first published 2013
© 2013 by John Wiley & Sons, Ltd

Wiley-Blackwell is an imprint of John Wiley & Sons, formed by the merger of Wiley's global Scientific, Technical and Medical business with Blackwell Publishing.

Registered office:
John Wiley & Sons, Ltd, The Atrium, Southern Gate, Chichester, West Sussex, PO19 8SQ, UK

Editorial offices:
9600 Garsington Road, Oxford, OX4 2DQ, UK
The Atrium, Southern Gate, Chichester, West Sussex, PO19 8SQ, UK
111 River Street, Hoboken, NJ 07030-5774, USA

For details of our global editorial offices, for customer services and for information about how to apply for permission to reuse the copyright material in this book please see our website at www.wiley.com/wiley-blackwell.

The right of the author to be identified as the author of this work has been asserted in accordance with the UK Copyright, Designs and Patents Act 1988.

Library of Congress Cataloging-in-Publication Data
Boyd, Claire.
   Clinical skills for nurses / Claire Boyd.
      p. ; cm. — (Student survival skills series)
   Includes bibliographical references and index.
   ISBN 978-1-118-44877-9 (pbk. : alk. paper) — ISBN 978-1-118-44876-2 (epub) — ISBN 978-1-118-44875-5 (epdf) — ISBN 978-1-118-44874-8 (emobi)
   I. Title. II. Series: Student survival skills series.
   [DNLM: 1. Nursing Care—methods—Handbooks. WY 49]
   610.73—dc23   2012047379

A catalogue record for this book is available from the British Library.

Wiley also publishes its books in a variety of electronic formats. Some content that appears in print may not be available in electronic books.

Cover image courtesy of Visual Philosophy
Cover design by Visual Philosophy

Set in Trade Gothic Light 9/12pt by Aptara Inc., New Delhi, India
Printed and bound in Malaysia by Vivar Printing Sdn Bhd

1 2013

Contents

Preface

Clinical Skills for Nurses is designed to assist the student healthcare worker in the field of clinical skills. All exercises are related to practice and the healthcare environment, from the acute hospital setting to the community, covering both adult and paediatric care.

The book looks at 12 clinical skills, requested by students like you, and gives a quick, snappy introduction to these skills in a non-threatening manner for you to gain a brief understanding and overview. You can then build on this foundation. For the present you may be permitted only to observe some of the skills that are covered, but that does not stop you from watching them being performed. This will be preparation for the day when you will be expected, often after a formal training event, to undertake them with your own patients.

I talk about 'patients' but the book applies to service users in the community setting as well. The paediatric nurse has not been forgotten, with information given throughout that incorporates this branch of nursing.

The book uses many activities and questions to check your understanding, and is laid out in a simple-to-follow, step-by-step approach. Each chapter ends with with a Test your knowledge section to relate everything learned to practice. The aim of this book is to start the individual on a journey through many healthcare-related exercises to build confidence and competence; from day one to qualification, and beyond. It has been compiled using quotes and tips from student nurses themselves; it is a book by students for students. I just wish a book like this had been around when I did my nursing training!

Claire Boyd
Bristol
October 2012

Introduction

Hello. My name is Claire and I am a Practice Development Trainer in a large NHS Trust. Let me tell you something about me: during one of my own clinical placements as a student nurse I was working in a doctor's surgery and was invited to observe a minor surgical procedure, namely a mole removal. The room was very small and hot and as the doctor cut into the skin on the lady's stomach, sounding very much like someone cutting into a cabbage, I felt very queasy. I was invited to take a closer look after the mole had been removed. I fainted while standing up, with my head laid down on the lady's stomach, and my nose in the mole crevice. At first the doctor and practice nurse thought how vigilant I was, wanting to take such a close look at the surgical site, until they realised I had fainted, whereby I was dumped unceremoniously to one side on the floor and the patient soothed. Every time I cut into a cabbage and hear that noise I am taken back to my training days and remember this incident with huge embarrassment.

There will be many tears and much laughter throughout your own training and this book attempts to help you along the way, helping you to gain some of the skills you require to become an excellent health carer, something we should all be striving to achieve.

The table below shows the skills that student nurses may, or may not, be able to perform during placements and at which stage of their training. Note that *this list varies from trust to trust and from university to university*. These skills may also not be transferable between trusts, so students will need to access their own university's and trust's guidelines and only work within those parameters, to avoid breaking vicarious liability.

Clinical skill	Nurse training, year 1	Nurse training, year 2	Nurse training, year 3	Qualified
Performing observations	✓	✓	✓	✓
Male urethral catheterisation	No	No	No	✓
Female urethral catheterisation	✓	✓	✓	✓
Bowel care	✓	✓	✓	✓
Tracheostomy care	No	✓	✓	✓
Point of care	✓	✓	✓	✓
Blood transfusion	Collection of blood only	Collection of blood only	Collection of blood and monitoring	✓
Venepuncture	No	✓	✓	✓
Peripheral cannulation	No	No	No	✓
Early patient assessment and response	✓	✓	✓	✓
Intravenous therapy	No	No	No	✓
Basic life support	✓	✓	✓	✓

Skills may also require different degrees of supervision, and again this may vary between trusts and educational providers. The four degrees of supervision are:

1 *Direct supervision not required once assessed as competent by a mentor.* Examples: measurement and application of TED stockings, ECG recording.
2 *Always to be performed under direct supervision.* Examples: replacing an inner tracheostomy tube; checking, calculating dosage and administering non-controlled drugs through the following routes: inhalation, PO, PR, PV, SL, topical, eyes, ears, enteral feeding tubes, IM and SC injections.
3 *May be performed but only after completing a Trust training programme and required competencies.* Examples: venepuncture, blood glucose monitoring.
4 *Must not perform this skill under any circumstances until qualified.* Examples: removal of CVP line, insertion of a fine-bore nasogastric tube for feeding purposes.

The registered nurse retains accountability at all times for assessing an individual student's knowledge, attitude and competence. But it is up to the student to check what skills they can perform, with:

- the mentor,
- trust policy,
- the university decision-making framework.

With some skills students may only be able to undertake part of that skill. For example, in blood transfusion a student nurse may be permitted (according to local trust policy and university guidelines) to go and collect the blood from the pathology laboratory (after training and being deemed competent). Only in the third year, when about to qualify, may this same student nurse be permitted to undertake a patient's observations while the blood is being transfused. A student nurse can *never* put up the blood products on the patient, not until they are qualified, and usually two nurses are involved in this process for safety reasons.

This book will therefore look at clinical skills you may or may not be permitted to be involved in, but which have been included to cover the wide range of students reading this book (from day one of your nurse training to the very last day). It is hoped that it will take you through your training, through all the tears and laughter this will involve (and there will be tears along the way!), giving you a good grounding in these clinical skills. They have been chosen by students themselves: they are the skills *they* wanted included in this book. I hope that I have made the writing style informal but brief, as though I am sitting beside you in your clinical placement. All the answers to the activities, questions and `test your knowledge' exercises can be found at the back of the book.

Acknowledgements

First thanks go to the many wonderful student nurses I have taught in all the clinical skills. Believe me when I say that learning has been a two-way process. Again, as in other books in the Student Survival Skills Series, it is their tips and quotes that have made this book what it is.

Acknowledgements also go to North Bristol NHS Trust and to certain individuals in particular for making this book possible, namely Jane Hadfield (Head of Learning and Development), Dr Karen Mead (Lead Transfusion Practitioner), the Biochemistry Laboratory team, Nick Smith (Clinical Educator, High Dependency Unit) and the NBT tracheostomy working party, and all my friends and colleagues in the Staff Development Department.

Thanks also go to Magenta Styles, Executive Editor at Wiley-Blackwell, for first approaching me for this exciting project and then for her guidance and direction in writing this book. Catriona Cooper, Project Editor at Wiley-Blackwell and Dr Nik Prowse for his copy editing comments.

For Chapter 8, special thanks to BD Diagnostics (www.bd.com) for allowing reproduction of information and diagrams.

This book is dedicated to my loving family: my long-suffering husband Rob (for the photographs), Simon, Louise and David. Thank you for supporting me in this exciting project.

Chapter 1

PERFORMING OBSERVATIONS

Clinical Skills for Nurses, First Edition. Claire Boyd
© 2013 John Wiley & Sons, Ltd. Published 2013 by John Wiley & Sons Ltd.

LEARNING OUTCOMES

By the end of this chapter you will have an understanding of the theory and practice of performing respiration, temperature, heart rate and blood pressure clinical observations.

Performing observations of vital signs on patients is a fundamental healthcare task. Every time a set of observations are taken, valid consent must be obtained from the patient.

CONSENT

When a patient lacks the capacity to consent, as with all clinical skills, observations can be made if it is in the patient's best interests. This is part of the UK Mental Capacity Act 2005, which is an Act of Parliament. Its primary purpose is to provide a legal framework for acting and making decisions on behalf of adults who lack the capacity to make particular decisions for themselves.

The three key factors when testing for valid consent are:

- does the patient have enough information to make the decision?
- does the patient have enough capacity to make the decision?
- has the patient made a free choice?

All three tests must be met for you to have obtained valid consent.

OBSERVATION CHARTS

Observation charts have changed considerably over time, since the introduction of the Early Warning Score, whereby we are able to assess our patients and care for them before their condition becomes critical. We will look at Early Patient Assessment and Response (EPAR) in Chapter 10, but for now we will start with the basic vital signs, looking at how to perform these tasks.

All patients admitted to hospital should have a 'manual' set of essential observations recorded; this is known as a **baseline**. Any changes to this norm will trigger action. Of course, the patient could be so ill as to present with a set of abnormal readings, but it is still useful to monitor the patient on admission so that we can see when progress is being made with the patient's condition.

BODY TEMPERATURE

Body temperature is measured using a calibrated clinical electronic thermometer or tympanic thermometer. In children's nursing, 'smart-material' tempo dot thermometer strips are often used (see overleaf). Mercury glass thermometers are used very rarely in hospitals today. It is considered best practice to document the temperature recording on the observation chart as a solid dot, connecting these dots with a straight line. This is the same procedure as for documented recordings of all vital signs.

The sites for recording body temperature are described below.

- *Oral:* the thermometer is placed in the posterior sublingual pocket, situated at the base of the tongue.
- *Axilla:* the thermometer is placed in the centre of the armpit, with the patient's arm lying across their chest. The same site should be used for all recordings; that is, do not change armpits.
- *Rectum:* a special thermometer is inserted at least 4 cm into the anus of an adult, or 2–3 cm in infants. This provides the most accurate reading of all sites. Rectal temperature readings are usually about 1°C higher than readings taken in the ear.
- *Ear:* to take a temperature reading in the ear a device known as a tympanic membrane thermometer, which is covered with a disposable cuff, is inserted snugly into the ear canal (Figure 1.1). These devices use

GLOSSARY

Tympanic membrane

The membrane in the eardrum separating the outer and middle ears.

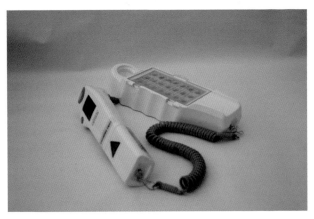

Figure 1.1 A tympanic membrane thermometer

infrared light to measure body temperature. The same ear should be used each time for consistent results. Some clinical areas have reconfigured the display screen to show the oral temperature, but the device must still be placed in the ear.

Single-use plastic-coated 'smart-material' strips are also used, often in paediatric care, which have heat-sensitive dots that change colour to indicate the temperature. The strip can be placed across the forehead or in the mouth as shown in Figure 1.2.

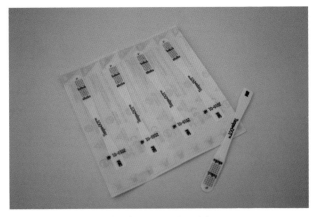

Figure 1.2 Tempo dot thermometer strips

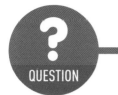

Question 1.1   What are the reasons for recording an individual's body temperature? List five, if you can.

Body Temperature Physiology

Body temperature is usually maintained between 36 and 37.5°C. A body temperature well above the normal range (41°C) is called **hyperthermia** and can result in convulsions. A temperature below normal temperature (35°C) is called **hypothermia** (Table 1.1).

Table 1.1 Hyperthermia and hypothermia

Condition	Possible causes
Hyperthermia	Heat stroke, malignancy, stroke or central nervous system damage
Hypothermia	Environmental exposure, medication and exposure of body and internal organs during surgery

Pyrexia is defined as a rise in body temperature, above the normal, usually caused by a viral or bacterial infection. Lay person's terminology for this is 'having a temperature' (see Table 1.2).

Table 1.2 Pyrexia

Low-grade pyrexia	Normal to 38°C
Moderate- to high-grade pyrexia	38–40°C
Hyperpyrexia	40°C and above

Procedure to Obtain the Temperature Using a Tympanic Membrane Thermometer

In many clinical areas, staff *must* have undertaken training in the use of this equipment.

1 Explain and discuss the procedure with the patient. Gain consent.
2 Wash your hands.

3   Check which ear is being used for the reading.
4   Remove thermometer from the base unit and ensure the device is clean (Figure 1.1).
5   Place a disposable probe cover on the probe tip.
6   Gently place the probe tip in the ear canal to seal the opening, ensuring a snug fit.
7   As soon as device indicates (usually by bleeping) remove it from the ear.
8   Press the release/eject button on the device to remove the probe cover.
9   Replace the thermometer in its base unit.
10 Record the reading on the patient's observation chart.

Documenting a Temperature Reading on an Observation Chart

Let's look at the observation chart (Appendix 1). Just for the moment we will keep it simple (in Chapter 10 we go into the EWS or Early Warning Score system in more depth). You will notice that each of the sections for vital signs (temperature, respiratory rate, etc) are colour-coded. At the bottom of this document you will see what score each of the colours represents. Let's say our patient has a temperature of 36.5°C, this is in the white section of the chart and scores zero. If this same patient had a score of 39.0°C it would be in the peach-coloured section and would generate a score of 2. Without going into any more detail yet, here are the actions we would perform with each score:

0–1	Continue with routine observations.
2–3	Report this information to the nurse in charge immediately.
4 and above	Re-check score. Inform the nurse in charge. Request a medical review within 15 minutes. Record the action taken.

Of course, we would usually do a full set of observations and tot up the scores for all the vital signs to get our final EWS score for that time.

BLOOD PRESSURE

Blood pressure is the force extended by the blood as it flows through the blood vessels, and increases with age, weight gain, stress and anxiety. Normal range for an adult is usually considered to be from 100/60 to 140/90 mmHg. The first figure is known as the **systolic** reading and the second figure is the **diastolic** reading. Although we record both figures on our observation chart, it is only the systolic reading that generates a score. Table 1.3 lists some of the terms you may hear in relation to the blood pressure reading.

Table 1.3 Terms related to the blood pressure reading

Normotension	Blood pressure within normal range
Hypotension	Blood pressure lower than normal range
Hypertension	Blood pressure higher than normal range

Of course, we should never lose sight of the fact that we are all individuals and have our own 'normal' range for the vital signs.

Blood pressure equipment

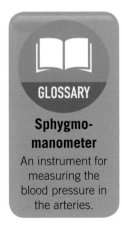

GLOSSARY

Sphygmo-manometer

An instrument for measuring the blood pressure in the arteries.

Increasingly electronic sphygmomanometers (also known as automatic or oscillometric machinery; see Figure 1.3) are being used to monitor blood pressure, but these may not achieve the same level of accuracy as manual sphygmomanometers (also known as aneroid sphygmomanometers; see Figure 1.4). This is especially so in certain disease states, such as arrhythmias, pre-eclampsia and certain vascular diseases. Staff using these machines should be trained and assessed on how to use them correctly.

Automated blood pressure machines should also not be used on patients with irregular heart rates or on patients with movement disorders, such as Parkinsonian tremors. These patients' blood pressure recordings should be taken using a manual aneroid sphygmomanometer and stethoscope, which you will be shown how to use during your nurse training.

Medics may occasionally request that patients have a 'lying and standing' blood pressure recording, and this is exactly how it sounds: taking the blood pressure first while the patient is

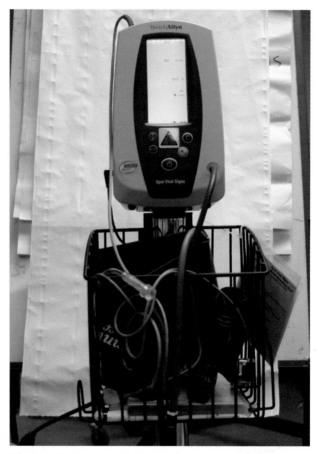

Figure 1.3 An automated blood pressure machine

lying down, then when standing. Beware that the patient may experience postural hypotension and feel dizzy when standing.

Which arm was used to record the blood pressure should be documented in the care plan, due to variations in reading and consistency. Blood pressures should not be taken from a patient's arms that are affected by arteriovenous fistulae, paralysis or breast surgery, or in which intravenous (IV) lines are situated.

Blood pressure cuffs should be the appropriate size to fit the patient, to ensure accurate measurement. The cuff

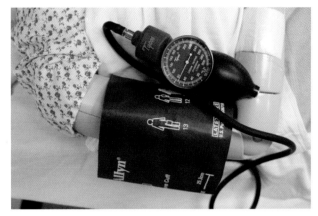

Figure 1.4 An aneroid sphygmomanometer

should cover 80% of the circumference of the upper arm or appropriate limb and should be checked for latex if using on a latex-sensitive individual. Many latex-free cuffs are now available. These cuffs should also be wiped clean between patient use to avoid cross-contamination from patient to patient.

Some clinical areas may still have mercury sphygmomanometers, but these are being used much less frequently today due to the dangers of mercury spillage.

Activity 1.1

Our patient has had his blood pressure taken hourly. Plot these recordings for the last 5 hours on a copy of the observation chart shown in Appendix 1. Do any of these readings generate a score?

130/70 mmHg
140/70 mmHg
170/74 mmHg
190/90 mmHg
202/90 mmHg

Procedure to Obtain Blood Pressure Using an Aneroid Sphygmomanometer and Stethoscope

You will be shown how to perform this skill during your training, so don't worry if you don't understand the procedure yet. You will need plenty of practice.

1 Wash your hands.
2 Explain procedure to the patient and gain their consent.
3 Gather equipment and clean the stethoscope with an alcohol wipe.
4 Assist the patient into a comfortable position with the arm to be used resting on a firm surface.
5 Roll up the patient's sleeve, making sure this is not too tight; otherwise this will lead to an inaccurate recording. It may be best to take the arm out of the sleeve if this may be the case.
6 Position the sphygmomanometer at approximately heart level, ensuring the dial is set at zero.
7 Apply the blood pressure cuff approximately 3–5 cm above where the brachial artery can be palpated (located at the inner side of the biceps). Connect the cuff tubing to the manometer tubing and close the valve to the inflation bulb.
8 Palpate the radial pulse and inflate the cuff until the pulse disappears. Inflate a further 20 mmHg. Release the valve slowly and note when the radial pulse returns. Allow the air to escape from the cuff.
9 Palpate the brachial pulse: Place the stethoscope over the brachial pulse site and inflate the cuff 20 mmHg above the previous reading.
10 Release the valve slowly.
11 When the first pulse is heard, the reading should be noted: *this is the systolic blood pressure.*
12 Continue to deflate the cuff and the pulse will change to a muffled sound until it finally disappears. The reading should be noted: *this is the diastolic blood pressure.*

13 Completely deflate the cuff and remove it from the patient's arm.
14 Clean the stethoscope and cuff.
15 Document the blood pressure recordings and report any abnormalities.
16 Wash your hands.

HEART RATE

Heart rate varies according to age. We can see what the heart rate is by using the pulse rate, which is measured by palpating an artery that lies close to the surface of the body. The radial artery in the wrist is often the area of choice due to its accessibility. Normal pulse rates per minute are displayed in Table 1.4.

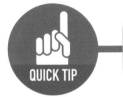

QUICK TIP

Heart rate can be felt by feeling the pulse points, so sometimes it is referred to as the pulse rate.

Table 1.4 Pulse rates at various ages

Age	Approximate range (beats per minute)
Newborn	120–160
1–12 months	80–140
12 months–2 years	80–130
2–6 years	75–120
6–12 years	75–110
Adolescent	60–100
Adult	60–100

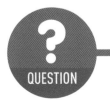

QUESTION

Question 1.2   What are the sites of the major pulse points and where are they located on the body?

The sites of the major pulse points can be viewed in the Figure 1.5.

The pulse should be taken for one full minute, assessing for rate, regularity and volume. Patients with a known or suspected irregular heart rate should have a manual reading taken each time this observation is performed.

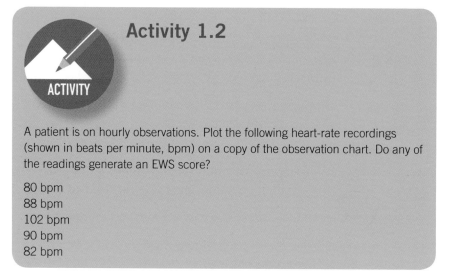

Activity 1.2

ACTIVITY

A patient is on hourly observations. Plot the following heart-rate recordings (shown in beats per minute, bpm) on a copy of the observation chart. Do any of the readings generate an EWS score?

80 bpm
88 bpm
102 bpm
90 bpm
82 bpm

An abnormally fast heart rate (over 100 beats per minute in adults) is known as **tachycardia**. This may be caused by raised body temperature, physical/emotional stress or heart disease, as well as certain drugs.

An abnormally slow heart rate (less than 60 beats per minute) is known as **bradycardia**. This may be caused by low body temperature and certain drugs. Very fit athletes also tend to have low pulse rates.

Procedure to Obtain a Pulse Reading

1 Wash your hands.
2 Explain the procedure to the patient and gain their consent.
3 Locate the radial artery by placing the second and third fingers along it and press gently. Some nurses prefer to use three fingers for this.

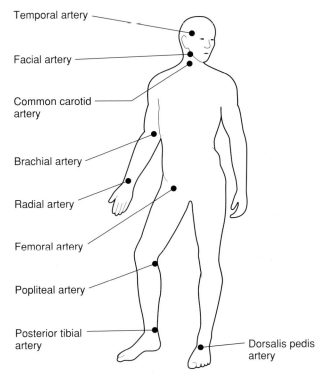

Figure 1.5 Pulse points (Smith and Roberts, 2011)

4 Count the pulse for 60 seconds, assessing for rate, regularity and volume.
5 Document the recordings and report any irregularities or abnormalities.
6 Wash your hands.

RESPIRATIONS

On the Bristol Observation Chart, the respiratory rate section is at the top, showing how crucial this recording is. A change in a patient's respiratory rate is a sensitive predictor of deterioration, and can be a precursor to an adverse event, such as a cardiac arrest, up to 4 hours prior to its occurrence. Trends in respiratory rate on a chart are therefore very important.

The respiratory system supplies the body with oxygen and removes the carbon dioxide through the rhythmic expansion and deflation of the lungs. Each respiration consists of an inhalation, exhalation and pause.

Ventilation is the act of breathing, with air moving in and out of the respiratory tract. Ventilation is under **involuntary control**, being dependent on the respiratory centre in the medulla oblongata and pons varolii, which are situated at the top of the brain stem.

Ventilation is also under **voluntary control** and is regulated through the central nervous system (CNS). The CNS enables individuals to maintain conscious control over their breathing rate.

It is for this reason we should not let patients know when we are counting the rise and fall of their chest (monitoring the **respiratory rate**) as they can alter their natural readings.

The respiratory rate is the number of breaths per minute. Normal respiratory rates vary according to age, with the accepted normal ranges displayed in Table 1.5.

Table 1.5 Respiratory rate in various age groups

Age group	Approximate range (breaths per minute)
Healthy adults	14–20
Adolescents	18–22
Children	22–28
Infants	30 or more

A good respiratory assessment should be assessed over one full minute, and includes looking, and reporting on:

- the *rate* of breathing: regular or irregular,
- the *depth* of breathing: normal, shallow or deep,
- the *patient's colour*: pink, flushed, cyanosed,
- the *sounds* and *ease* of breathing: effortless, laboured, noisy, abnormal.

Abnormal patterns of breathing are described in Table 1.6.

Table 1.6 Abnormal patterns of breathing

Pattern	What to look for
Dyspnoea	Difficult, laboured breathing. Shoulders are often raised, nostrils dilated and veins visible in the neck.
Cheyne–Stokes	There is a gradual increase in the depth of respiration followed by a gradual decrease and then a period of no respiration (apnoea). This syndrome is associated with end-of-life care.
Kussmaul's respirations	There is an increased rate and depth of respiration with panting and long grunting expirations. Associated with lobar pneumonia.
Stertorous respirations	Noisy respirations caused by secretions in the trachea or bronchi. May be due to partial airway obstruction.
Stridor	A high-pitched noise heard on inspiration which is caused by laryngeal obstruction: this is a medical emergency.

The next activity looks at the terminology you will come across in relation to respirations.

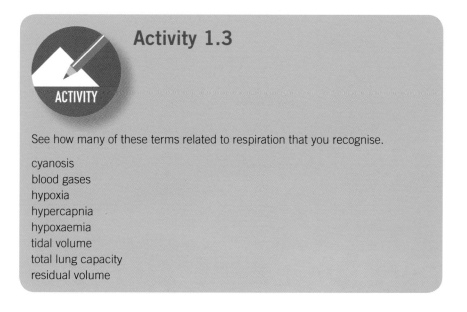

Activity 1.3

ACTIVITY

See how many of these terms related to respiration that you recognise.

cyanosis
blood gases
hypoxia
hypercapnia
hypoxaemia
tidal volume
total lung capacity
residual volume

Procedure to Obtain a Reading for Respiratory Rate

1 Ensure the patient is relaxed and not aware that you are assessing their respirations.
2 Count the respiratory rate and assess the rate, depth and ease of breathing and patient's colour (for cyanosis) for one full minute.
3 Document the recordings and report any abnormal findings.

NEUROLOGICAL OBSERVATIONS

A full neurological assessment is conducted using the Glasgow Coma Scale (GCS), which is outlined in Chapter 10 (see Figure 10.1). The GCS looks at the patient's level of consciousness, pupillary activity, motor function, sensory function and their vital signs, with each test equating to a score. We will look at this in more depth in Chapter 10, where you will be shown how to use the tool.

Many clinical areas use the **AVPU** assessment tool. If you look at the Bristol Observation Chart and the Neuro Response section you will see the following:

A = Alert
V = Responds to voice or a change in the verbal response
P = Responds to painful stimuli
U = Unresponsive

Only the alert recording does not generate a trigger or score. If the patient is V, P or U we would need to measure their GCS and inform the nurse in charge.

Procedure for Obtaining an AVPU Recording

Simply approaching our patient and talking to them will tell us if they are alert (A) or responding to voice (V). If we are required to give them a painful stimulus, this is usually conducted by performing a 'trapezium squeeze'.

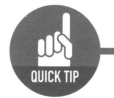

The trapezium squeeze: using the thumb and two fingers, hold 5 cm of the trapezium muscle, where the neck and shoulder meet, and twist.

OXYGEN SATURATION

Oxygen saturation (SpO_2) is routinely measured with a pulse-oximetry machine, after training and assessment to use this machinery.

Red blood cells contain haemoglobin molecules that bind with oxygen to form oxyhaemoglobin. Pulse oximetry works on the principle that blood saturated with oxygen is a different colour to deoxygenated blood. The clean probe, which is placed on a finger, contains a light source and detector which shines through the tissues of the body to obtain the oxygen saturation reading.

The pulse oximeter will not display a correct estimate of the oxygen saturation unless the machine is able to accurately capture the patient's pulse reading. The user should always check the patient's manual pulse against the waveform displayed by the machine.

Pulse oximeters will not give accurate measurements if the patient is peripherally compromised or wearing nail varnish, as this interferes with the light source on the probe. Bright or fluorescent room lighting may also interfere with the light transmission on the probe. Pulse detection on the probe may be interfered with by patient movement (such as Parkinsonian movement disorders), rigors or shivering.

Due to the limitations with this machinery, the pulse oximeter should not replace either the manual respiratory rate or pulse measurement.

Oxygen saturation is recorded on the Bristol Observation Chart (in the section marked SpO_2). The *target* oxygen saturation should have been identified by a medic, and should include whether it is to be attained with or without oxygen therapy. In other words, we are looking to see if the patient's oxygen saturation is within the acceptable range, as stated by a medic. The normal arterial oxygen saturation is approximately 95–98%.

TEST YOUR KNOWLEDGE

Go back to the Bristol Observation Chart and input these observations from a patient. What is this patient's Early Warning Score? What would be your actions?

Respiratory rate: 30 breaths per minute
Oxygen saturation, SpO_2: 95%
Blood pressure: 192/74 mmHg
Heart rate: 110 beats per minute
Neurological response: alert
Temperature: 38.4°C

KEY POINTS

- Obtaining valid consent.
- Using the Bristol Observation Chart.
- Performing vital-sign observations of temperature, blood pressure, heart rate, respiration, neurological indicators and oxygen saturation.

Chapter 2

MALE URETHRAL CATHETERISATION

Clinical Skills for Nurses, First Edition. Claire Boyd
© 2013 John Wiley & Sons, Ltd. Published 2013 by John Wiley & Sons Ltd.

LEARNING OUTCOMES

By the end of this chapter you will have an understanding of the theory and practice of performing the clinical skill of male urethral catheterisation.

Urinary catheterisation can be defined as 'the insertion of a special tube into the bladder, using aseptic technique, for the purpose of *evacuating* or *instilling* fluids' (Dougherty and Lister, 2011).

Catheters are hollow tubes with an eyelet at one end (which sits in the bladder) to facilitate drainage of urine along and out of the tube. Indwelling urethral catheters have a balloon to hold the tube in place in the bladder (see Figure 2.1).

Catheters are measured in Charrières (abbreviated to Ch), which is the circumference of the catheter in millimetres, equivalent to three times the diameter. Therefore a 12 Ch catheter has a diameter of 4 mm. Most adult male urethral catheterisations are performed using a 12 Ch or a 14 Ch catheter. The scale is also sometimes called the French scale, abbreviated to Fr.

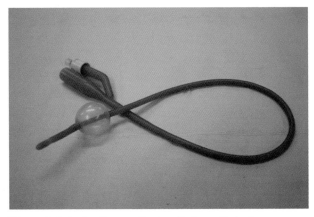

Figure 2.1 Indwelling urethral catheter, with balloon inflated

POLICIES AND PROCEDURES

When performing the clinical procedure of urinary catheterisation, your own employer's policy should be read and cross-referenced to other policies in your area, such as those on:

- universal infection-control precautions,
- hand hygiene,
- disposal of waste,
- handling and transportation of pathology specimens policy,
- collection and transport of clinical specimens,
- consent: assessment of mental capacity and determining best interests (documented),
- use of latex,
- chaperones.

Reading these policies and procedures is to protect the patient, and you, to ensure that you do not break 'vicarious liability'. Tilley and Watson (2008) define it as:

> …the principle by which a practitioner's employer will take liability for the actions and omissions of the employee as long as they are acting within their job description and boundaries approved by the employer.

So we must follow the safety measures (i.e. the policies and procedures) that have been put in place, and act within our job description and employer's boundaries.

WHY IS URINARY CATHETERISATION PERFORMED?

Prior to undertaking urethral catheterisation, we need to conduct a thorough assessment of our patient. Usually, urinary catheterisation is undertaken under three main categories: for drainage, for investigation or for instillation.

Drainage

- Bladder outflow obstruction
- Acute or chronic retention
- Detrusor under activity
- Pre- and post-pelvic surgery, e.g. lower urinary tract surgery
- Accurate measurement of urine output
- Determination of residual volume
- Comfort for the terminally ill
- Prevention of skin breakdown
- Relief of incontinence when no other means is practicable

Investigation

- To obtain an uncontaminated urine specimen if unobtainable by non-invasive methods
- In urodynamic investigations
- X-ray investigation

Instillation

- To irrigate the bladder
- To instil medication, e.g. chemotherapy

The assessment should also consider:

- cognitive status,
- patient's ability to manage the catheter, if appropriate,
- carer availability to support catheter care, if appropriate,
- tissue viability and preservation of skin integrity.

If a patient lacks the mental capacity to consent to the procedure it may still be carried out in their best interests, and documented accordingly.

FLUID OUTPUT

When I first did my nurse training, we talked constantly about meeting the '30 mL per hour' target as we thought this was the magic figure for urine output that all patients needed to achieve for us to know that their renal function was not impaired. We now know this is not true: a 107 kg man will not have the same output as a 50 kg older woman! What were we thinking? Thank goodness for evidence-based nursing! Let me show you what this means in practice.

Let me show you an example...

e.g.
EXAMPLE

Using the old system, we'd expect a 70 kg person to produce 30 mL of urine each hour. In 24 hours this equates to 720 mL (30 mL × 24 hours = 720 mL). This does not take into account the person's body weight, however.

Now, if we use the formula:

$$\text{Urine output} = 0.5 \text{ mL/kg/h}$$

This does take into account the person's body weight. So, for a 70 kg woman, inputting this body weight into the formula, we find that daily urine output would be expected to be:

$$0.5 \text{ mL} \times 70 \text{ kg} \times 24 \text{ hours} = 840 \text{ mL}$$

This makes a huge difference: 120 mL. Pulling this into practice, we thought that 720 mL was satisfactory when in effect this output was too low, as a person of this size should be producing 840 mL every day.

But even using the formula does not give us the whole picture, as medical conditions such as hypotension may mean that the kidneys are not being fully perfused. This patient may have a congested cardiac condition and be prescribed a diuretic medication, such as furosemide. Many patients call these pills 'water tablets' as they cause increased micturition. This woman may be critically ill and be experiencing 'peripheral shutdown', or become dehydrated. In short, we need to look at the patient holistically: this means looking at the whole picture and not using a formula like the one given above in isolation.

HIGH-RISK PROCEDURE

Urinary catheterisation is classed as a high-risk procedure, as it is very often the mode for micro-organisms to enter the human body.

The UK Department of Health's Saving Lives campaign was a delivery programme to reduce healthcare-associated infections such as methicillin-resistant *Staphylococcus aureus* (MRSA), and includes reducing the incidence of urinary tract infections (UTIs). The programme provided tools for Acute Trusts to make significant reductions to infection rates of MRSA bloodstream infections by 2008. The high impact areas were:

- High Impact Intervention no. 1: preventing the risk of microbial contamination,
- High Impact Intervention no. 2: central venous catheter care,
- High Impact Intervention no. 3: preventing surgical site infection,
- High Impact Intervention no. 4: care of ventilated patients,
- High Impact Intervention no. 5: urinary catheter care.

Many Trusts have adapted these tools to collect data on infections in these core areas and report their infection rates to the Department of Health. Trusts then incur fines if the numbers are higher than they should be. In the case of urinary catheter care there is a weekly audit of every patient in the clinical area with a urinary catheter *in situ*, and infections are reported. So, although the campaign has now officially been completed, the infection-rates audit are still being maintained.

Now, when we catheterise a patient in an NHS hospital we need to collect data and report every incidence of catheter-associated UTI (or CAUTI). Urinary catheterisation is High Impact Intervention no. 5, due to the fact that:

- more than 40% of all hospital-acquired infections are CAUTIs,
- there is a daily risk rate of 5–8% of developing a CAUTI,
- 20–30% of catheterised patients develop bacteriuria; 2–6% of these develop UTIs,
- 4% of these UTI patients develop bacteraemia and 13–30% of them die,
- 80% of all CAUTIs are caused on insertion.

Male catheterisation has always been considered as an 'advanced role' separate from female catheterisation. This is due to males having a prostate gland, which could potentially be punctured during the process of inserting the catheter.

As men head towards their 'three score years and ten' (that is, age 70), the prostate naturally enlarges. This is a very vascular process, meaning if the gland does get punctured the patient could bleed to death.

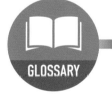

GLOSSARY

Vascular
Relating to or supplied with blood.

PERSONAL CARE AND THE NEED FOR STRICT ASEPSIS

As a catheter tube is a 'foreign body' within the body we need to take particular care with the patient's personal care, so as not to introduce microbes into their system. One of the entry points for these microbes is the join between the catheter tube and the attached drainage bag. It is for this reason that the connection between the catheter and the urinary drainage system must not be broken, except when renewing the catheter bag.

Also, practitioners must decontaminate their hands using the six-step hand-wash technique with water and soap or alcohol gel, and wear non-sterile gloves before manipulation of the catheter system.

Meatal and suprapubic site care must be carried out with unperfumed soap and water daily, or as required if build-up of secretions is evident. I can't tell you the number of times I have pulled back a foreskin and found a substance akin to cream cheese. This is due to a build-up of the bacteria that we do not want to travel up the catheter tubing, into the bladder, to cause a systemic catheter-associated infection.

Perfumed soap may cause irritation to this sensitive area. Remember, not all men have a foreskin; for those with a foreskin, this should be eased down gently over the catheter after cleaning, in order not to cause a paraphimosis.

Talcum powder and creams should not be used around catheter sites, as these may cause microbe colonisation by travelling up the catheter tube. As we wipe the catheter tubing, we wipe away from the body, down the tube.

The drainage bag should be positioned above the floor but below bladder level to prevent reflux or contamination. Obviously this is not the case with 'belly bags' which are worn around the waist. All drainage bags should be hung either on a catheter stand or a bed-hanger stand. They should never be dragged along on the floor, as it will cause the bag to pick up germs.

During catheter insertion, strict asepsis must be maintained. Dressing packs for this procedure come in many different varieties. Check to see if your pack contains sterile gloves, or whether you will need to put a pack onto your dressing trolley.

ANATOMY AND PHYSIOLOGY

Before we can begin to learn a new clinical skill we need to have some knowledge of the basic anatomy and physiology associated with the skill.

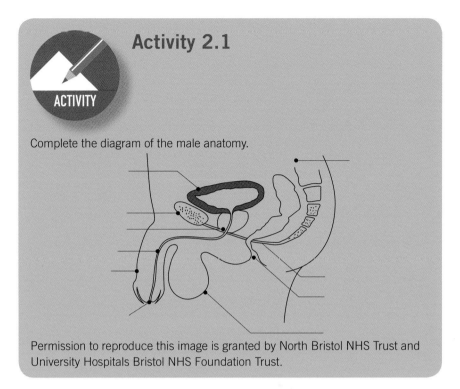

Activity 2.1

Complete the diagram of the male anatomy.

Permission to reproduce this image is granted by North Bristol NHS Trust and University Hospitals Bristol NHS Foundation Trust.

The main function of the kidneys is to act as a filtration system and to maintain bodily fluid, electrolyte and acid/base balance. These organs also play a part in synthesis of vitamin D and the detoxification of free radicals and drugs.

The ureters are tubular organs than run from the renal pelvis to the bladder. They are approximately 25–30 cm in length and 5 mm in diameter in adults. Their purpose is to transport urine from the renal pelvis into the bladder.

The bladder is a hollow muscular organ that stores urine. It is usually able to hold between 350 and 750 mL of urine in adults. In the inner floor of the bladder is the nerve supply, or trigone. These sensory nerves travel to the brain and pass on signals that the bladder requires emptying. Motor nerves are then activated to inform the detrusor muscle and internal and external sphincters to allow urine to flow out from the bladder along the urethra.

In males, the urethra is approximately 15–20 cm in length. It has to pass through the prostate gland before reaching the penis. The prostate is a vascular organ that produces fluid that forms part of the semen.

The Prostate

Tests to determine an enlarged prostate usually take the form of a digital examination, whereby two gloved and lubricated fingers are inserted up the man's anus to feel for the prostate. The prostate should be walnut-sized, relatively soft and slightly spongy.

A screen for prostate-specific antigens (PSAs) can also be taken, in the form of a simple blood test. However, although these tests are becoming more accurate they may give a false positive if the patient has been massaging his scrotum, recently had sexual intercourse and/or has recently had a rectal examination, all of which cause a rise in PSA levels.

Presently the definitive test in the UK for prostate malignancy is a biopsy. Recent research by the Institute of Cancer Research UK has looked at the link between male finger length and the risk of developing prostate cancer. The finding is that those with longer ring fingers are more at risk. Here's how to assess this:

1   measure from the crease at the bottom of the ring finger to the tip (this is the finger next to the little finger),
2   measure from the crease at the bottom of the index finger to the tip (this is the finger next to the thumb),
3   men with longer index fingers than ring fingers are significantly *less likely* to get prostate cancer.

It's all to do with the amount of the hormone testosterone a baby is exposed to in the womb. Being exposed to less testosterone equates to a longer index finger, and a reduced chance of getting prostate cancer in later life.

CATHETERISATION

There are three types of urinary catheterisation.

1 *Intermittent*: the lubricated catheter tube is inserted into the bladder, up the urethra, to drain urine every 4–6 hours. The tube is withdrawn each time and disposed of. A clean technique is performed. Those performing this on themselves are taught how to perform this skill and do require will power, dexterity and good cognitive function. This method of catheterisation can give individuals independence and control over their own bodies. It used to be called intermittent 'self-catheterisation' but as many carers now perform the technique it is now commonly known as clean intermittent catheterisation (or CIC).

2 *Urethral*: here, the catheter is inserted up the urethra and a balloon is gently blown up at the bladder end with approximately 10 mL of water (or however much water is required for a particular catheter). The catheter is then secured in place. Urethral catheters can be left *in situ* over the longer term (days or months), so subsequently have higher incidences of infection. At the end of the catheter tubing a drainage bag needs to be in place to collect the urine. Some individuals may not wish to use a drainage bag but instead have a valve, which works like a tap to drain the urine from the bladder, along the catheter tubing and out through the valve. It is not certain why indwelling catheterisation began to be used more frequently than self-catheterisation, but an advantage of this method of catheterisation is that it can be used over the course of long surgical procedures and when individuals are having bed rest, if deemed appropriate. This is also known as indwelling urethral catheterisation (URC), as the catheter remains in place.

3 *Suprapubic*: this is where the catheter is inserted through the anterior abdominal wall into bladder, whereby a stoma is created. A dressing is initially applied around the stoma but can be removed after

3–5 days, as warmth creates a higher incidence of infection. The wound should be observed for infection and over-granulation. An advantage of this method of catheterisation is that it can be used if urethral catheterisation is not feasible due to trauma, etc. In addition, suprapubic catheterisation leaves the individual's genitals free for sexual activity. This is also known as indwelling suprapubic catheterisation (SPC), as the catheter remains in place.

EXCLUSION CRITERIA FOR URETHRAL CATHETERISATION

Only specialist healthcare personnel should undertake urinary catheterisation on the following categories of individuals:

- within 48 hours of prostate surgery,
- those who have a history of urethral stricture,
- patients with a history of bacteraemia associated with catheterisation (unless the patient has been given appropriate antibiotic prophylaxis),
- those with symptomatic UTI (unless the patient has adequate antibiotic cover),
- patients with a priapism.

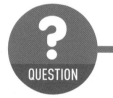

QUESTION

Question 2.1   What is a urethral stricture?
Question 2.2   What is a priapism?

CATHETER MATERIAL AND SELECTION

Indwelling urethral catheters came in a variety of materials and designs, depending on the rationale for insertion and insertion time. A balloon is inflated to keep the catheter in place in the bladder. A rule of thumb is that the smallest-possible catheter should be chosen to maintain drainage.

Catheters are usually categorised in one of three time scales, depending on how long the catheter is expected to be in place, with the catheter material reflecting this:

short term (1–14 days),
short to medium term (2–6 weeks),
medium to long term (6 weeks to 3 months).

- *PTFE-/silver-coated catheters*: these are usually inserted for up to 28 days. They are soft, but this allows crust formation. Teflon-coated or silicone (PTFE) elastomer-coated catheters have a latex core. This reduces urethral irritation. Silver-alloy coated catheters are thought to reduce bacterial colonisation in the longer term. Note: PTFE = Polytetrafluoroethylene
- *Hydrogel-coated latex catheters*: these are used for up to 12 weeks. They are well tolerated by the urethral mucosa, causing little irritation to the mucosal lining. They are reported to be resistant to bacterial colonisation and encrustation.
- *All-silicone catheters*: these are used for up to 12 weeks. They have a wider lumen, which is crescent- or D-shaped, but due to being rigid they may be more uncomfortable. They are the only sort suitable for patients with latex allergy.
- *Hydrophilic catheters*: these are for intermittent use. They are lubricated for ease of insertion, and come in a variety of designs. Figure 2.2 shows a selection of these catheters.

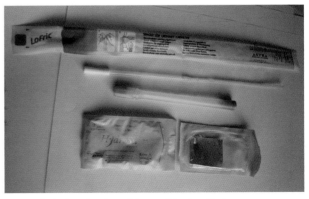

Figure 2.2 A selection of intermittent catheters

Whichever catheter is selected, all catheters should be stored flat in their original boxes, and in a cool place. They should never be stored tied with rubber bands as this can bend the catheter and distort the water channel.

CATHETER LENGTH AND DESIGN

Catheters come in three lengths:

* standard (or 'male' length), 40–44 cm,
* female length, 23–26 cm,
* paediatric length, 30 cm.

Figure 2.3 shows a standard-length and a female-length catheter.

The UK National Patient Safety Agency (NPSA; a Department of Health watchdog) issued an alert stating the dangers of inserting a shorter, female-length catheter

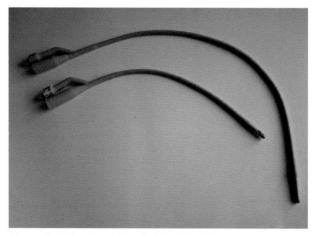

Figure 2.3 Standard-length (40–44 cm) and female-length (23–26 cm) catheters. Note that in many care settings only standard-length catheters are now used.

into a male and the damage this could cause when the balloon is inflated in the urethra rather than the bladder. The NPSA reported that in one 12 month period there were 114 incidents where female catheters were inserted into male patients. All experienced severe pain, some degree of haematuria, penile swelling or retention. Seven of these insertions caused significant haemorrhage, with two believed to have led to acute renal failure, and two to impaired renal function. It was due to this alert that many care settings removed the shorter-length catheters and now only insert the standard length into all patients (male and female).

> Adult urinary catheters are manufactured in two lengths: female length (20–26 cm), and standard length (40–45 cm). The use of standard length catheters in females poses no safety issues, as the shorter female length is designed for dignity issues when wearing skirts rather than trousers. However, if a female length catheter is accidentally used for a male, the 'balloon' inflated with sterile water to retain the catheter will be within the urethra, rather than the bladder, and can then cause severe trauma. (National Patient Safety Agency 2009)

Catheters are also available in designs other than with the standard round tip. This is to resolve particular problems associated with urinary catheterisation. For example, a Tieman-tipped catheter has a curved tip with up to three drainage eyes for greater drainage. Some patients may experience an output of urine with large amounts of debris and/or clots, so a larger catheter with larger eyelets or multiple eyelets may be used.

REMOVING THE CATHETER

There must be a daily review of the need for the catheter with a view to removing it as soon as possible.

Catheters should be removed following assessment of the individual's ongoing condition and in consultation with the individual and the multi-disciplinary team responsible for their care. The balloon will need to be deflated in order to allow the catheter tube to be pulled out through the urethra. The balloon valve must never be cut off. If difficulty is experienced during this process of deflation, assistance must be sought immediately.

When deflating the balloon to remove the catheter, just attach a syringe to the balloon valve on the catheter tube and allow the balloon to self-drain. *Do not aspirate* (i.e. draw back) the syringe as this pulls the mucosal wall into the catheter eyelet and may cause damage. With silicone catheters the balloon takes longer to drain, so you do need to be patient, but it only takes only a matter of moments in most cases. The longer the catheter has been in place, the longer the balloon will take to deflate.

After removal, fluid intake and output must be monitored carefully to ensure the bladder is emptying efficiently and that there are no episodes of incontinence.

DRAINAGE BAGS AND SECURING DEVICES

As the urine flows from the catheter tubing, a drainage device needs to be attached. These come in a variety of designs, such as leg bags for ambulatory patients, where the bag is attached to the patient's leg.

At night, a 'night bag' can be attached to a leg bag or other drainage day bag to collect larger volumes of urine (Figure 2.4). Night bags can be attached to a frame and these may be further attached to the bed frame. In the morning the night bag is detached, leaving the leg or day bag in place. Always remember to close the tap first before detaching the night bag, otherwise the urine will pour all over your shoes! When emptying these bags a closed system must be maintained, so as not to expose the patient to microbial contamination.

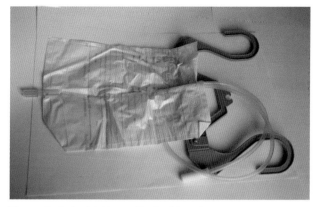

Figure 2.4 A night bag attached to a frame

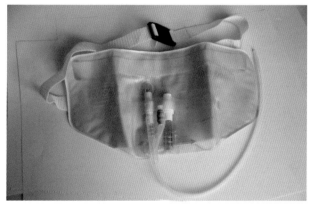

Figure 2.5 A catheter 'waist' drainage bag

Some individuals prefer to use a waist 'belly bag', which is actually just as the name suggests: it is worn around the waist, much like a 'bum bag'. It works on the principle of venous pressure pushing the urine upwards into the waist bag. Figure 2.5 shows one of these systems.

Leg bags are usually changed every 5–7 days, and belly bags every 28 days.

Whichever drainage bag has been selected, bags should be stabilised and secured (Figure 2.6). This is to prevent

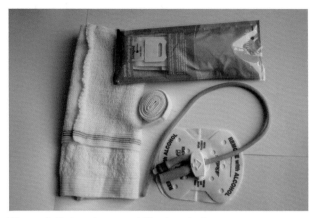

Figure 2.6 A catheter stabilisation devices

movement and pulling of the catheter tube, which in turn may cause trauma. Stabilisation may be maintained with the use of T-straps, aqua-sleeves or Statlock stabilisation devices. A Statlock stabilisation device is a strap-free device which locks a Foley catheter in place. The device is attached to the inner leg much like a plaster and is changed every 7 days.

Patients, often in acute care, may require a unometer, which is a diuresis-measuring system whereby acute urine output measures can be obtained.

Some individuals may prefer to use a catheter valve, which mimics normal bladder function (Figure 2.7). This is a valve that the individual opens intermittently to drain the bladder and which eliminates the need for a drainage bag. A valve usually gets replaced after 7 days.

Latex

Only latex-free catheters can be inserted into individuals with latex sensitivity, otherwise they could experience a full-blown allergic reaction causing anaphylaxis. Individuals known to have a sensitivity to certain foodstuffs, such as kiwi fruit, avocados and bananas, will

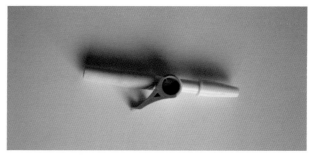

Figure 2.7 A catheter valve device

also need to avoid anything containing latex, as these foods contain the same proteins as latex and could cause a reaction.

Latex-sensitive patients will also need to receive their care with latex-free gloves in order to avoid a reaction.

Lubrication

Much has been written on the subject of the lubrication to be used when inserting the catheter. Many areas use lignocaine based lubricants, with anaesthetic properties. However, due to the contra-indications to these products, especially concerning patients with certain cardiac arrhythmias, hypertension, hepatic problems and epilepsy, etc., many areas have gone back to using water-based lubrication, such as KY jelly. It is important to find out the practice in your area.

Antibiotic cover

Again, much has been written about the use of prophylactic antibiotics in routine catheterisation. The use of antibiotics in these circumstances has not been supported by evidence-based research, and indeed the high incidence of increased resistance to antibiotics has been attributed to their overuse in the past.

Some areas ask those prescribing antibiotics for routine catheterisations to consult a microbiologist to see if it is warranted. As nurses, we may be the ones expected to administer this antibiotic, either orally or by injection, so it is important to check the rationale for the prescription.

PROBLEMS ASSOCIATED WITH CATHETERISATION

The act of inserting a urethral catheter may present many complications to the patient, immediately and over the duration of its placement. Some of these problems may include:

- urethral trauma resulting in infection and possible septicaemia/renal failure/death,
- formation of false urethral passage,
- bladder perforation,
- traumatic removal of catheter with balloon inflated,
- urinary tract infection and possible septicaemia/renal failure/death,
- by-passing of urine around catheter,
- urethral stricture formation,
- meatal tears,
- encrustation and bladder calculi,
- urethral perforation,
- pain,
- bleeding,
- bladder spasm,
- reduced bladder capacity,
- catheter blockage,
- latex sensitivity,
- altered body image,
- difficulties with sexual relations.

One of the main considerations associated with urinary catheterisation is infection. Ninety per cent of catheterised individuals will get a UTI within 4 weeks of a urethral catheterisation.

Other problems associated with catheterisation are:

- catheter-associated urinary tract infection (CAUTI),
- tissue damage,
- pressure necrosis,
- abscess formation,
- discomfort,
- loss of dignity,
- paraphimosis.

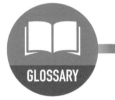

GLOSSARY

Paraphimosis

A paraphimosis is a tightening of the foreskin behind the glans penis. The foreskin is unable to be drawn back, causing pain and swelling to the penis.

When bladder hyper-irritability occurs, a medic may prescribe diazepam to stop the urethral going into spasm. The carer may also need to consider inserting a smaller catheter of different material as this is what may be causing the irritability to the urethral and leakage of urine to occur.

Good documentation must be performed when providing any clinical skill. In the case of catheterisation, certain information needs to be documented, such as:

- catheter type, length and size,
- batch number,
- manufacturer,
- amount of water instilled into the balloon,
- date and time of catheterisation,
- reasons for catheterisation,
- colour of urine drained,
- any problems negotiated during the procedure,
- a review date to assess the need for continued catheterisation or date of change of catheter.

If no urine drains, medical staff should be informed immediately. Ongoing care is mediated by use of a catheter care plan, an example of which can be viewed in Figure 2.8.

Urinary Catheter Care Plan

North Bristol **NHS**

Date of insertion: ....

Estimated date for removal or change:
....

Indication for catheter?

- Accurate fluid balance (critically ill?)
- Urine retention
- Major Surgery
- Other (please specify):
- Urinary tract haemorrhage
- Palliative
- Skin breakdown from incontinence

Please record actions each shift.
Please record in boxes below √ =yes × =no
Please record A/C for actions that are daily or weekly and have already been completed
Please initial after each review at the bottom of the care plan

Date	E	L	N	E	L	N	E	L	N	E	L	N	E	L	N	E	L	N	E	L	N
Action																					
1. **Hand hygiene** Before and after each patient contact																					
2. **Catheter hygiene** Clean catheter site at least once a day as per policy CP1e																					
3. **Drainage bag position** Above floor but below bladder level to prevent reflux or contamination and assist drainage																					
4. **Sampling (needle-free) aseptically via catheter port**																					
5. **Manipulation -Securing the catheter** Catheter secured using a fixation device using aseptic technique and comfortable for patient. Leg straps must be removed at night.																					
6. **Manipulation - Catheter drainage bag emptying** Empty at least twice daily. Gloves and apron must be worn. Clean container used every time. Decontaminate port before emptying. Avoid touching drainage tap. Decontaminate hands after taking gloves and apron off.																					
7. **Manipulation - Changing drainage bag** Urine drainage bags and valves must be dated and changed at least every 7 days.																					
8. **Catheter needed?** Review daily, remove as soon as possible																					
Please initial after each shift																					

SES. 22.12.10

Date	Variance	Sign

Guidance

Hand hygiene 5 moments
Before touching patient
Before clean. aseptic technique
After body fluid exposure
After touching patient
After touching patient surroundings

Sampling
Perform aseptically via the catheter port
Catheter manipulation (any action which involves touching the catheter system)
Examination gloves must be worn to manipulate a catheter, and manipulation should be preceded and followed by hand decontamination.
Maintain a closed system
Connection between catheter and drainage bag must not be broken except for good clinical reason e.g. changing drainage bag.
Single use non-drainable night bag may be used at night.
Recording
Record urinary output on fluid chart .if appropriate
Encourage good fluid intake.
Report poor output, (adequate output is 0.5 ml per kg of patient's body weight per hour e.g.33 mls if patient weighs 66 kgs.)
Report any changes in colour e.g. blood
Self management of hygiene & emptying
Following education and help if appropriate.
After removal of catheter
Ensure patient is within easy reach of a toilet or voiding receptacle.
Monitor intake and output, ensure patient is comfortable and feels that the bladder is empty after voiding.
Record episodes of incontinence.

For further information refer to: Policy for Adult Urethral Catheterisation and Supra-pubic Re-catheterisation Policy CP 1e

SES. 22.12.10

Figure 2.8 A urinary catheter care plan. Reproduced here with permission from North Bristol NHS Trust and University Hospitals Bristol NHS Foundation Trust

HOW TO TAKE A CATHETER SAMPLE OF URINE

A catheter sample of urine is abbreviated to CSU. A CSU should only be taken:

- to diagnose UTI if the patient has systemic signs or symptoms consistent with a urinary infection,
- as part of an MRSA screen when indicated,
- for culture before elective orthopaedic implant surgery,
- prior to defined urological procedures.

A CSU should not be taken just because:

- the urine is cloudy,
- the urine in the bag is 'dipstick-positive', meaning that a urinalysis test has been performed and the urine contains elements that should not be present, such as protein, ketones, blood, sugar, etc.,
- the catheter is blocked,
- the urine smells offensive.

A sample of urine should always be obtained via the sample port, and never the drainage bag itself. The sample should be obtained under aseptic technique

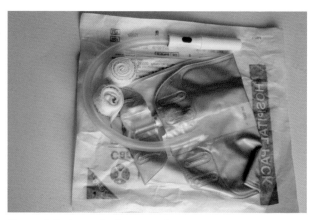

Figure 2.9 A needle-free sample port

and after the sample port has been cleaned. Many sample ports are now designed for syringes only, known as 'needle-free sample ports'; these are usually red (Figure 2.9). Some areas may still use needle-and-syringe sample ports, which may be coloured blue. However, these are more prone to causing needlestick injuries. Both these ports 'self-seal' after the sample has been obtained.

EMPTYING A DRAINAGE BAG

An apron and gloves should be worn for this procedure. Prior to opening, the tap on the drainage device should be cleaned with an alcohol wipe (and again after the procedure). After the urine has been collected, the collection device should be covered when taking it to the sluice or toilet for disposal.

If the individual has a fluid chart, remember to measure the volume of urine, and document this. Remove the apron and gloves and your wash hands with soap and water after each procedure.

How to empty a catheter drainage bag:

- empty the drainage bag frequently enough to maintain urine flow and prevent reflux,
- wash your hands,
- use a clean pair of non-sterile gloves,
- risk assess for need to wear face protection (goggles),
- before emptying, decontaminate the port with alcohol wipes,
- urine bags should not be emptied into plastic reusable jugs as this may cause cross-contamination,
- a separate and clean container should be used for each patient,
- take care not to let the catheter drainage port the touch sides of the container,
- after emptying the catheter bag the port should be decontaminated using alcohol wipes.

PROCEDURE FOR MALE URETHRAL CATHETERISATION

Now for the procedure of inserting the urethral catheter. Remember, it is usual to undertake this procedure after attending a study session and undergoing supervised practice before being deemed competent and confident to be able to perform the task. After the procedure it is considered best practice to give the patient an information booklet or sheet that explains the procedure.

If the patient consents, have a 'runner' to hand; that is, someone who needs to learn the ropes and who can collect any equipment required during the procedure. For example, you may drop a piece of equipment and need to replace it. Never leave your patient exposed, even for a moment.

Prior to catheterisation, the patient must have a good clean 'down below' with soap and water, so send them to the bathroom. Instruct them that, if they have a foreskin, they need to pull it back and wash underneath. Although we advocate self-care wherever possible, some patients may not be able to undertake this wash themselves, so we may need to take a bowl of warm water to the bedside and wash the patient ourselves. This wash is very important, as cleaning the meatus and penile shaft during the aseptic part with sodium chloride will not remove all the germs if the patient is very mucky down there.

The equipment

1	Sterile catheterisation pack	6	Appropriate catheter valve, and support accessories for catheter bag
2	Disposable and waterproof pad	7	Light source
3	Sterile and non-sterile gloves	8	Sterile water and syringe for the balloon. (if not included in catheter pack)
4	Appropriate size and length of catheter	9	Disposable plastic apron
5	Pre-packed sterile anaesthetic lubricating gel	10	Drainage bag and stand or holder if appropriate

11	0.9% Sodium chloride (Normasol sachet)	13	Information leaflet/booklet with contact name if appropriate
12	Alcohol hand rub		

Guidelines for male catheterisation

	Action
	Action
1	Explain and discuss the procedure with the patient. Gain consent.
2a	Screen the bed. Ensure good light source. Ask patient to shower or wash glans penis and scrotal area with soap and water in bathroom if able. Otherwise perform this task for the patient.
2b	Assist the patient to get into the semi-recumbent position with the legs extended.
2c	Do not expose the patient at this stage of the procedure. Ensure that the patient is warm.
3	Wash your hands using soap and water using the six-step hand-washing technique.
4	Clean and prepare the trolley, placing all equipment required on the bottom shelf.
5	Take the trolley to the patient's bedside, disturbing screens as little as possible.
6	Open the outer cover of the catheterisation pack and slide the pack onto the top shelf of the trolley.
7	Using an aseptic technique, open the supplementary packs. Open catheter into sterile receiver.
8	Remove cover that is maintaining the patient's privacy and position a disposable pad under the patient's buttocks and thighs.
9	Put on a disposable plastic apron and non-sterile disposable gloves.
10	Retract the foreskin, if necessary, and clean the glans penis with 0.9% sodium chloride (Normasol), moving from the meatus to the base of the penis.
11	Remove non-sterile gloves and clean hands using the six-step technique with alcohol gel. Put on sterile gloves.
12	Place the sterile sheet with the hole over the penis.
13	Warn patient of risk of stinging from anaesthetic gel. Squeeze a drop of the single-use anaesthetic gel onto tip of catheter and also cover the meatus with gel. Then squeeze the remainder of the gel into urethra.
14	Hold the penis with a piece of gauze firmly for 3–5 minutes.

15	Hold the penis (at approximately 65°) behind the glans, raising it until it is almost totally extended. Place the receiver containing the catheter between the patient's legs. Insert the catheter until urine flows and advance almost to the bifurcation.
16	If resistance is felt at the external sphincter, increase the traction on the penis slightly, and ask patient to cough and apply gentle, steady pressure on the catheter.
17	Gently inflate the balloon according to the manufacturer's instructions.
18	Withdraw the catheter slightly and attach it to a compatible valve or drainage system. Support the catheter by using a specifically designed support strap. Ensure that the catheter does not become taut when the patient mobilises.
19	Ensure that the glans penis is clean and reposition the foreskin.
20	Make the patient comfortable. Ensure that the area is dry.
21	If this is the first catheterisation, after 20 minutes measure the amount of urine drained.
22	Dispose of equipment and gloves in a clinical waste bag and seal the bag before moving the trolley.
23	Draw back the curtains.
24	Dispose of clinical waste bag into a clinical waste bin.
25	Wash and dry hands thoroughly as per the six-step procedure and document all information.

TEST YOUR KNOWLEDGE

1 What are the three main methods of catheterisation?
2 Give an advantage of each.
3 Give a disadvantage of each.
4 Name six complications associated with urethral catheterisation.
5 Name two of the exclusion criteria for urethral catheterisation.
6 How often should the following equipment be changed?

catheter valve
catheter drainage bags
catheter 'belly bags'

7 What is best practice in catheter care? Is the use of talcum powder and cream recommended?

8   After catheterisation, what information should be recorded in the patient records?

9   Where are CSUs collected from the drainage bags?

10 After a catheter drainage bag has been emptied using an aseptic technique, what should the port be decontaminated with?

KEY POINTS

- Reasons why urinary catheterisation are performed.
- Catheter care.
- Exclusion criteria for urethral catheterisation.
- Drainage bags.
- Problems associated with urinary catheterisation.
- Procedure for male urethral catheterisation.

Chapter 3
FEMALE URETHRAL CATHETERISATION

Clinical Skills for Nurses, First Edition. Claire Boyd
© 2013 John Wiley & Sons, Ltd. Published 2013 by John Wiley & Sons Ltd.

WHY IS URINARY CATHETERISATION PERFORMED?

Female urinary catheterisation is performed for the same reasons as male urethral catheterisation – for drainage, investigations and instillations – with the added purpose of:

- emptying the bladder during childbirth.

ANATOMY AND PHYSIOLOGY

Before undertaking the clinical skill of female urethral catheterisation, we need to have knowledge of the female anatomy.

Activity 3.1

Complete the diagram of the female anatomy.

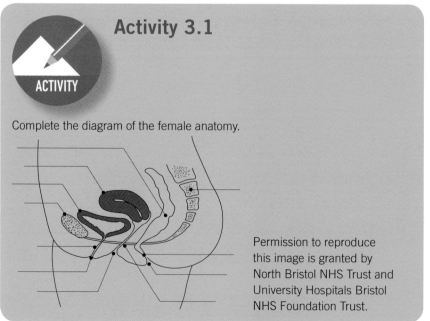

Permission to reproduce this image is granted by North Bristol NHS Trust and University Hospitals Bristol NHS Foundation Trust.

Female catheterisation can be trickier to perform than male catheterisation, as three orifices are quite close together. As a woman gets older everything appears to move 'south' (i.e. downwards) making finding the urethra, into which we must insert the catheter tube, more difficult to locate, especially if the patient is overweight. It is for this reason that very often the catheter tube is inadvertedly inserted into the vagina. In this case, as no urine will be flowing out of the catheter, it is best to leave the tube in place until another tube is inserted, hopefully this time into the urethra. Only then do we remove the first tube that went into the vagina.

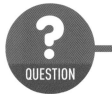

QUESTION

Question 3.1   Why would you leave the catheter tube in place if you know it is not in the urethra?

Pelvic Floor

The pelvic floor, which males also have, is a set of muscles that stretches like a hammock from the pubic bone in the front to the bottom of the backbone. These firm, supportive muscles help to hold the bladder, womb and bowel in place. The muscles are firm and kept slightly tense to stop urine leakage from the bladder or leakage of faeces from the bowel.

When we pass urine, or have a bowel motion, the pelvic floor muscles relax to facilitate this. Afterwards they tighten again to prevent further movement or leakage.

Over time, the pelvic floor muscles can become weak and sag due to a variety of reasons, such as childbirth, the menopause and hormonal changes, lack of exercise, or obesity, as extra weight puts extra strain on these muscles. As the pelvic floor becomes weaker, urine leakage and/ or faecal leakage may then occur, being more evident when women laugh, sneeze or exercise. This can be very embarrassing.

As with any muscle, 'if you don't use it, you'll lose it'. Pelvic floor exercises can strengthen these muscles and have been found to be particularly effective for stress incontinence (a type of urinary incontinence), improving or even stopping leakage of urine as the muscles become stronger over time.

As health professionals, part of our role is in education, and we may need to inform our patients on techniques to improve the pelvic floor. One technique is shown below.

- This pelvic floor exercise can be done sitting down, or standing up. Imagine yourself sitting on the toilet passing urine. Now imagine yourself stopping the flow of urine: really 'pull' upwards and squeeze and stop it. You may find this hard to start with. Some people are able to manage the technique of 'going up' in stages: much like a life going up floors! As you practise this exercise, you can try holding for a few seconds and then relaxing and letting go.
- Now, if you are not already sitting, sit down, with your knees slightly apart. Imagine you are trying to stop yourself passing wind from the bowel. Really squeeze and lift the muscle around your back passage. You should feel the skin around the back passage being pulled up and away from the chair and you should feel the muscle move, but your buttocks and legs should not move.

You can do these exercises at any time, in any place and unless you pulled some strange faces while you were doing them, no one need know! Also don't worry if you could not feel the muscles very well, as over time the pelvic floor will strengthen and tighten and you will gain more control over them.

Another good exercise to strengthen the pelvic floor, as long as you don't have back, hip, or knee pain and discomfort, are pelvic tilts:

- stand with you feet 30 cm apart, with your knees slightly bent. Now rotate hips in a clockwise circular movement. Do this for approximately 10 minutes every day.

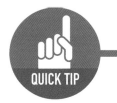

QUICK TIP

Avoid high-impact-type physical exercises, as these may weaken the pelvic floor muscle. Yoga, pilates, swimming, cycling and belly dancing are considered 'good' exercises to do if you are experiencing bladder weakness.

FLUID BALANCE

Fluid balance is an essential tool in determining hydration. If there are problems with fluid balance then it may indicate warning signs that the patient is acutely or potentially ill. If fluid balance is not monitored correctly then such signs can be missed, resulting in:

- late referral and missed opportunities,
- unexpected deterioration,
- prolonged stay in hospital,
- in some cases, death.

NOTE: weighing incontinence pads may not be a problem when recording fluid balance, but weighing sheets may well be. Therefore, practise estimating amounts of any wet sheets on beds.

PERSONAL CARE

Good hygiene procedures must be maintained to prevent infection when a patient has a catheter *in situ*. Daily, or more frequent, washing must be undertaken. The gold standard for washing is good, old fashioned soap and water. The catheter tube should be wiped downwards, away from the body. Sometimes a patient may ask for 'a sprinkling' of talcum powder. This can cause infection as the talc may transgress into the bladder, up along the tubing, and the patient should therefore be dissuaded. However, if a patient has mental capacity and you have informed them of the rationale for its non-use, and they still wish to have some, then you will need to document this fact.

PROCEDURE FOR FEMALE URETHRAL CATHETERISATION

Catheter types are shown in Figure 2.2. Remember that the shorter, female-length catheters should now not be used on men or women, following an alert by the NPSA (National Patient Safety Agency 2009). Only standard-length catheters are now used in many care settings (see Chapter 2 for more details).

The Equipment

1	Sterile catheterisation pack	8	Sterile water and syringe for the balloon (if not included in catheter pack)
2	Disposable and waterproof pad	9	Disposable plastic apron
3	Sterile and non-sterile gloves	10	Drainage bag and stand or holder if appropriate
4	Appropriate size and length of catheter	11	0.9% Sodium chloride (Normasol sachet)
5	Pre-packed sterile anaesthetic lubricating gel	12	Alcohol hand rub
6	Appropriate catheter valve, and support accessories for catheter bag	13	Information leaflet/booklet with contact name if appropriate
7	Light source		

Guidelines for Female Catheterisation

	Actions
1	Explain and discuss the procedure with the patient. Gain consent.
2a	Screen the bed. Ensure good light source. Ask the patient to shower or wash vulval area with soap and water in bathroom if able. Otherwise assist patient to perform this task.
2b	Assist the patient to get into the supine position with the legs extended.
2c	Do not expose the patient at this stage of the procedure. Ensure the patient is warm.
3	Wash hands using soap and water using the six-step hand-washing technique.

4	Clean and prepare the trolley, placing all equipment required on the bottom shelf.
5	Take the trolley to the patient's bedside, disturbing screens as little as possible.
6	Open the outer cover of the catheterisation pack and slide the pack onto the top shelf of the trolley.
7	Using an aseptic technique, open the supplementary packs. Open catheter into sterile receiver.
8	Remove cover that is maintaining the patient's privacy and position a disposable pad under the patient's buttocks and thighs.
9	Put on a disposable plastic apron and non-sterile disposable gloves.
10	Assist the patient to get into the supine position with knees bent but apart, hips flexed and feet together.
11	Separate the labia minora so that the urethral meatus is seen. If there is any difficulty in visualising the urethral orifice due to vaginal atrophy and retraction of the urethral orifice, consider re-positioning the patient, for example by raising the patient's buttocks, and ensure the lighting is good.
12	Clean both the labia and around the urethral orifice with 0.9% sodium chloride (Normasol) using single downward strokes.
13	Remove non-sterile gloves and clean hands using the six-step technique with alcohol gel and put on sterile gloves.
14	Warn the patient of the risk of stinging from anaesthetic gel. First, squeeze a drop of the single-use anaesthetic gel to cover the meatus. Then squeeze the gel into the urethra and discard the tube. Wait for 3–5 minutes.
15	Place the catheter, in the sterile receiver, between the patient's legs.
16	Introduce the tip of the catheter into the urethral orifice in an upward and backward direction. Advance the catheter until urine flows steadily.
17	Gently inflate the balloon according to the manufacturer's instructions; ensuring the catheter is draining properly beforehand.
18	Withdraw the catheter slightly and attach it to a compatible valve or drainage system.
19	Support the catheter by using a specifically designed support strap. Ensure that the catheter does not become taut when the patient is mobilising.
20	Make the patient comfortable. Ensure that the area is dry.
21	If this is the patient's first catheterisation, after 20 minutes measure the amount of urine drained.

TEST YOUR KNOWLEDGE

1   What is the first thing you must do prior to performing a urethral catheterisation?
2   Where does the pelvic floor sit?
3   What is considered the 'gold standard' when proving catheter care?
4   Why is female urinary catheterisation performed?

KEY POINTS

- The pelvic floor.
- Female anatomy and physiology.
- Fluid balance.
- Procedure for female urethral catheterisation.

Chapter 4
BOWEL CARE

Clinical Skills for Nurses, First Edition. Claire Boyd
© 2013 John Wiley & Sons, Ltd. Published 2013 by John Wiley & Sons Ltd.

Bowel care management includes the assessment and observation of a patient's stools and seeking and/or providing treatment for any dysfunction. Bowel care management may also include the clinical procedures of digital rectal examination (DRE), administration of enemas and/or suppositories, digital removal of faeces (DRF) and digital rectal stimulation (DRS), and risk assessments and contra-indications for these procedures, including autonomic dysreflexia.

Many patients are embarrassed to discuss their bowel function so we are talking about a very sensitive issue. A poor patient, with limited mobility, is very often expected to 'open their bowels' on a commode, next to their bed, with just a flimsy curtain between them and their neighbour. Mix into the equation the change of diet, change of environment and change of medication – including analgesia, etc. – it is no wonder that some patients get constipated. Worse still is when a patient contracts a hospital-acquired infection (or HAI) such as C. diff (short for *Clostridium difficile*), which causes diarrhoea!

To start off we first need to look at the basic anatomy and physiology of the bowels and some key basic principles.

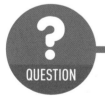
QUESTION

Question 4.1   What do you think are the five main functions of the bowel?

ANATOMY AND PHYSIOLOGY OF THE BOWELS

Information from the lower bowel and brain is conveyed via sympathetic (lumbar) and parasympathetic (sacral) nerve roots: the autonomic

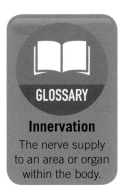

GLOSSARY

Innervation

The nerve supply to an area or organ within the body.

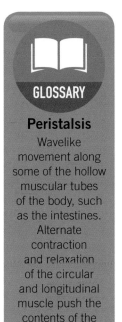

GLOSSARY

Peristalsis

Wavelike movement along some of the hollow muscular tubes of the body, such as the intestines. Alternate contraction and relaxation of the circular and longitudinal muscle push the contents of the tube forward.

nervous system. These are the pudendal nerves (from the external genital organs) which carry fibres from the sacral nerves S2–S4 to the pelvic floor muscle and descending colon and rectum.

The sympathetic innovation comes from thoracic nerves T9–T12, and it is these that keep the anal sphincter closed. The parasympathetic nervous system relaxes the anal sphincter when we need to defecate. This voluntary control usual starts at age 18 months, when we learn to control this movement to defecate in the right place and at the right time.

What we eat enters the mouth, thus beginning the digestive process, and travels down the oesophagus and into the stomach (see Figure 4.1). From here the food is broken down by digestive enzymes and the vitamins, proteins, water, etc. are digested and absorbed to be utilised by the body. The intestinal contents are moved along by peristalsis, taking approximately 3–5 hours to travel along the small intestine. You may have heard the expression 'gut motility' to describe this movement process.

The matter then travels up the ascending large colon, along the transverse large colon and down the descending large colon, into the rectum to the anal canal and out the anus.

If the faeces are not expelled for some time, they will become hard and more difficult to pass, resulting in constipation (Box 4.1 gives the diagnostic criteria for constipation).

Diarrhoea may be **acute** (usually lasting less than 2 weeks) and may be caused by an infection, or **chronic** (lasting more than 2 weeks) and may be due to inflammatory bowel disease (Box 4.1 gives the definition of diarrhoea).

Any bowel dysfunction may have a profound effect on an individual – both physiologically and/or psychologically and will require a sensitive approach to treat.

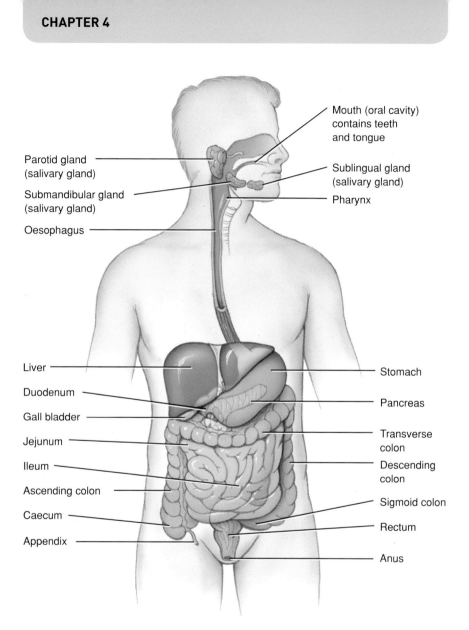

Mouth (oral cavity) contains teeth and tongue

Parotid gland (salivary gland)

Sublingual gland (salivary gland)

Submandibular gland (salivary gland)

Pharynx

Oesophagus

Liver

Stomach

Duodenum

Pancreas

Gall bladder

Jejunum

Transverse colon

Ileum

Descending colon

Ascending colon

Caecum

Sigmoid colon

Rectum

Appendix

Anus

Figure 4.1 The digestive system. Reproduced from Peate and Nair (2011) with permission

Box 4.1 Definitions of constipation and diarrhoea

Constipation may be defined when two or more of the following are present:

- straining for at least a quarter of the time,
- lumpy hard stool for at least a quarter of the time,
- a sensation of incomplete evacuation for at least a quarter of the time,
- two or fewer bowel movements in 1 week.

Diarrhoea may be defined as: the frequent evacuation or the passage of abnormally soft or liquid faeces.

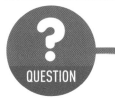

QUESTION

Question 4.2   What do you think are the causes of bowel dysfunction? List five.

ASSESSMENT

When assessing any bowel dysfunction we need to establish the patient's normal bowel pattern, as they may normally produce 'loose' stools, so this is 'normal' for them. Any dysfunction to the normal pattern will then need to be investigated, and for a good assessment will need to look at:

- history of onset (is it linked to any lifestyle or emotional changes? Has the patient recently travelled abroad?),
- normal bowel pattern,
- present bowel pattern (also look at consistency and colour of stool and any blood present),
- stool chart recordings (using the Bristol Stool Chart; see overleaf),
- diet and fluid intake (any changes? Is the patient adequately hydrated?),
- medication (any changes?),
- understanding/mental capabilities (has our patient become confused?),
- skin breakdown (any changes to perianal or peristomal integrity?),
- mobility (any changes?),
- physical assessment.

THE BRISTOL STOOL CHART

The Bristol Stool Chart was developed by Dr Ken Heaton at the University of Bristol and can be used to evaluate the effectiveness of treatments for various diseases of the

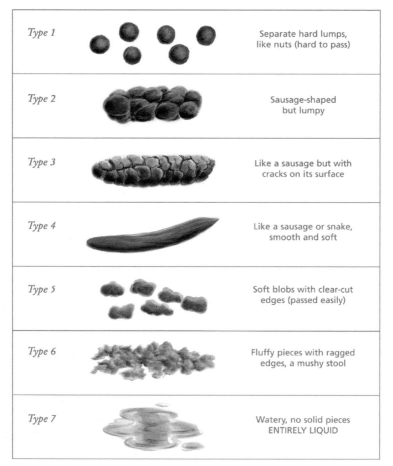

THE BRISTOL STOOL FORM SCALE

Type 1	Separate hard lumps, like nuts (hard to pass)
Type 2	Sausage-shaped but lumpy
Type 3	Like a sausage but with cracks on its surface
Type 4	Like a sausage or snake, smooth and soft
Type 5	Soft blobs with clear-cut edges (passed easily)
Type 6	Fluffy pieces with ragged edges, a mushy stool
Type 7	Watery, no solid pieces ENTIRELY LIQUID

Figure 4.2 The Bristol Stool Chart. Permission to reproduce this image is granted by North Bristol NHS Trust and University Hospitals Bristol NHS Foundation Trust

bowel. It is also used as an assessment tool to monitor our patients' bowels before any problems occur (Figure 4.2).

Type 1 and Type 2 stools may be difficult to pass due to constipation. We could advise our patients who produce these stools to increase their fibre intake and hydration, if their medical condition allows. This caution is required because increasing dietary fibre (e.g. adding bran to the diet) may lead to faecal loading, slow transit time, increased flatus and increased pain for patients with conditions such as irritable bowel syndrome.

Type 3 and Type 4 stools are considered to be the easiest stool to pass, and are therefore the 'ideal' stool.

Type 5, 6 and 7 stools are tending towards diarrhoea, with Type 7 possibly resulting in dehydration, electrolyte imbalance and malnutrition, as well as abdominal pain/cramping and perianal skin breakdown. Patients with ileostomies and colostomies will also need to change their appliances more frequently, possibly causing peristomal skin breakdown.

So you see, this assessment tool, which is now used worldwide, is an important part of the whole patient assessment process, as once we have established a dysfunction, treatment can commence. Table 4.1 shows a few of the medications that may be used in the care of bowel dysfunction.

Table 4.1 Medications used in bowel care

Medication type	Information
Acute diarrhoea	
Antimotility drugs	Antimotility drugs may be used in the management of uncomplicated acute diarrhoea in adults, but not in young children.
Codeine phosphate: oral	Tolerance and dependence may occur with prolonged use.
Loperamide hydrochloride: oral	Used in the treatment of acute diarrhoea in adults and children over 4 years of age.
Morphine: oral	Causes sedation; risk of dependence.

(continued)

Table 4.1 *(Continued)*

Medication type	Information
Constipation	
Laxatives	Laxatives may be used in patients with constipation, after it has been established that the constipation is not secondary to an underlying undiagnosed condition. They may be prescribed as an enema or to be taken in oral form.
Bulk-forming	Bulk-forming laxatives relieve constipation by increasing faecal mass, stimulating peristalsis: Ispaghula Husk, Fybogel, Ispagel orange.
Stimulant laxatives	Stimulant laxatives increase intestinal motility. Excessive use can cause diarrhoea: Bisacodyl is an oral medication or presented in suppository format; Docusate Sodium, oral; glycerol, suppository; Senna, oral.
Faecal softeners	Enemas containing arachis oil (ground nut/peanut oil) lubricate and soften impacted faeces to promote a bowel action: arachis oil, enema.
Osmotic laxatives	Osmotic laxatives increase the amount of water in the large bowel, either by drawing fluid from the body into the bowel or by retaining the fluid they were administered with: Lactulose, oral; Macrogols, oral powder; Movicol, oral.

A **suppository** is a preparation that may be inserted into a body cavity, such as the rectum or the anus, in order to be absorbed to treat conditions such as constipation.

A **pessary** is the same, but goes into the vagina to treat conditions such as candidiasis (thrush). As well as a medication, a pessary may also be an instrument or ring to treat conditions such as a prolapsed womb.

An **enema** is fluid that is infused through a tube into the anus to remove faeces or to insert drugs into the rectum.

Many healthcare environments insist that staff administering medications via suppository or as an enema must have received bowel care training, and be assessed as competent to perform this clinical skill.

MEDICATION REVIEW

As part of the patient assessment process, and following an episode of constipation, faecal impaction or faecal incontinence, the patient's medications should be reviewed. This is due to the fact that many drugs have side effects that affect gut motility and stool consistency. The main groups are:

- broad-spectrum antibiotics,
- opioids,
- antidepressants,
- antimuscarinics,
- antihistamines,
- laxatives,
- antidiarrhoeals,
- iron preparations,
- obesity medication,
- antacids.

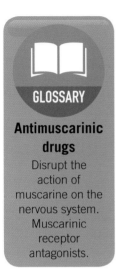

GLOSSARY

Antimuscarinic drugs
Disrupt the action of muscarine on the nervous system. Muscarinic receptor antagonists.

BOWEL CARE MANAGEMENT

Once all the initial assessments/treatments have taken place, further investigations may be deemed appropriate. This includes:

- digital rectal examination (or DRE),
- inserting enemas and/or suppositories,
- digital removal of faeces (or DRF),
- digital rectal stimulation (or DRS).

These clinical skills are usually **job-specific** (some healthcare assistants may be permitted, after training, to perform a DRE and insert enemas and suppositories) and **area-specific**, as in some clinical areas only registered nurses or assistant practitioners, operating department practitioners and medics can perform them. One of these areas is neuroscience, which includes neurosurgical and neuromedical wards, as these skills are very specialised in this category of patients, for reasons we will look at shortly (namely autonomic dysreflexia; see page 70).

Health carers who are able to perform these clinical skills, as with all clinical skills, are expected to abide by their local policies, and should be conversant with the following standards and guidelines:

Royal College of Nursing (2008a) *Bowel Care including Digital Rectal Examination and Manual Evacuation of Faeces. Guidance for Nurses.* Royal College of Nursing, London.

NICE (2007a) *Faecal Incontinence: The Management of Faecal Incontinence in Adults.* NICE Clinical Guideline 49. NICE, London.

In addition, check national guidelines, such as *Guidelines for Management of Neurogenic Bowel Dysfunction after Spinal Cord Injury* (produced by the Spinal Cord Injury Centres of the United Kingdom and Ireland, 2009) and Dougherty and Lister (2011).

EXCLUSIONS AND CONTRA-INDICATIONS

There are certain exclusions and contra-indications for performing bowel care management, listed below, as specialised care is required in these cases:

- where there is a lack of valid consent from a patient with capacity,
- the patient's medical team have given specific instructions that these procedures are not to take place,
- the patient has recently undergone rectal/anal surgery or trauma,
- rectal bleeding of unknown cause,
- malignancy of the perianal area,
- autonomic dysreflexia.

RISK ASSESSMENT

The carer should be confident and competent to perform any of these bowel management procedures and a full consultation between the patient and carer should be undertaken to clarify why the procedure is required. A full risk assessment should be performed, looking at specific issues, including:

- *health and safety*: latex allergies, peanuts, etc.,
- *documentation*: keep accurate documentation,
- *codes of conduct*: patient's dignity, high standards of care, etc.,
- *vicarious liability*: always follow employer's guidelines and procedures,
- *competence*: are you competent to perform this skill?,
- *consent*: cognitive ability, sufficient information, without coercion,
- *chaperone*: patient may wish to have a same-gender carer performing this activity (chaperone policies should be adhered to),
- *special precautions and contra-indications*: read patient's notes prior to undertaking the procedure and consult with medical staff and/or healthcare colleagues.

Circumstances When Extra Care is Required

It is important to gain all the information you can prior to undertaking these clinical skills. It is especially important to know the patient's medical history to be aware of circumstances when extra care is required, such as:

- active inflammation of the bowel, for example Crohn's disease,
- recent radiotherapy to the pelvic area,
- rectal/anal pain,
- obvious rectal bleeding,
- tissue fragility,
- if the patient has a history of abuse,
- if the patient has a history of allergies,
- the patient gains sexual satisfaction from the procedure.

Observations

When performing any of these bowel care management clinical procedures, it is considered best practice to perform vital-signs observations before, during and after the procedure. This is especially important in the neurological patient, and in others who may be considered at risk.

DIGITAL RECTAL EXAMINATION (DRE)

DRE is performed to:

- assess the presence of stool in the rectum, its amount and consistency,
- assess the need for rectal medication,
- evaluate the efficacy of interventions/medication,
- assess anal tone and contraction and its degree.

ADMINISTRATION OF ENEMAS AND/OR SUPPOSITORIES

Indications for the insertion of suppositories or enemas include:

- treatment of inflammatory bowel conditions,
- neurogenic bowel dysfunction, as part of a regular bowel management programme,
- evacuation of faecal matter from the bowel,
- spinal cord injuries, as part of a regular bowel management programme,
- drug administration as an alternative to the oral route, to be absorbed for systemic effect.

A DRE should be carried out to assess for faecal loading and for abnormalities including blood, pain and obstruction.

There has been much discussion about whether the blunt end of a suppository should be inserted first in order for it to be retained for longer. Research by Abd-el-Maeboud et al. (1991), published in *The Lancet*, stated that this method activates fewer nerve endings in the rectum, allowing it to be retained for longer; otherwise the bodily instincts tell us to push it out as it is a foreign object.

DIGITAL REMOVAL OF FAECES (DRF) IN ADULTS

DRF may be carried out where other bowel-emptying techniques have failed or are inappropriate, or when the patient has:

- faecal loading/impaction,
- incomplete defaecation,
- an inability to defaecate,
- neurogenic bowel dysfunction, as part of a regular bowel management programme,
- spinal cord injuries, as part of a regular bowel management programme.

When performing this clinical skill, it is important not to stretch the anus, so care should be taken to 'hook' the finger when performing this procedure. In spinal patients, a too-rigorous DRF can cause spinal shock.

DRF may be used as an acute intervention following DRE where other methods have failed, or as part of the patient's regular bowel management programme. DRF is defined as 'the insertion of a finger into the patient's rectum to evacuate the contents'. It should be avoided if at all possible since it is often distressing to the patient. Cultural and religious beliefs should be considered prior to performing this procedure (Royal College of Nursing 2008a).

DIGITAL RECTAL STIMULATION (DRS)

DRS may be carried out when the patient has:

- neurogenic bowel dysfunction, as part of a regular bowel management programme,
- spinal cord injuries with reflex bowel dysfunction, as part of a regular bowel management programme.

DRS is performed by rotating the finger *in situ* for 15–20 seconds, or until the internal sphincter relaxes. It should not be carried out for more than 1 minute at a time. This cycle can be repeated up to three times and an anaesthetic gel may be prescribed to ease the process.

AUTONOMIC DYSREFLEXIA

Autonomic dysreflexia (or ADR) is a syndrome unique to patients with **spinal cord injury** at the level of the sixth thoracic vertebra or above. It is a sudden, potentially lethal rise in blood pressure and is often triggered by acute pain or harmful stimulus, below the level of the injury. It should always be treated as a medical emergency; if left untreated, it can be fatal due to the risk of cerebral haemorrhage, seizure or cardiac arrest.

Autonomic dysreflexia only affects spinally injured patients. This is why the procedures discussed here can only be performed by experienced registered practitioners (registered nurses) in most clinical areas.

The condition arises as a result of an autonomic (sympathetic) reflex in response to pain or discomfort (noxious stimuli) perceived below the level of the lesion. The reflex creates a massive vasoconstriction below the level of the lesion causing a pathological rise in blood pressure that can be life-threatening if allowed to continue unchecked.

Advanced bowel care for this category of patients can only be performed by staff with specialised knowledge and skill.

Common Causes of Autonomic Dysreflexia

There are many triggers for this condition, such as:

- distended bladder (e.g. catheter blockage or bladder outlet obstruction),
- distended bowel (e.g. constipation, impaction or full rectum),
- ingrown toenail,
- fracture below level of the lesion,
- pressure ulcer,
- contact burn, scald or sunburn,

- urinary tract infections or bladder spasms,
- renal or bladder calculi,
- pain or trauma,
- deep-vein thrombosis,
- over-stimulation during sexual activity,
- severe anxiety.

Signs and Symptoms of Autonomic Dysreflexia

- Pounding, usually frontal, headache
- Severe hypertension (spinal cord-injured patients have a lower resting blood pressure)
- Slow pulse

One or more of the following:

- flushed appearance of the skin above the level of the injury,
- profuse sweating above the level of the injury,
- pallor above the level of the injury
- nasal congestion.

Treatment of Autonomic Dysreflexia

Under normal circumstances a tetraplegic person may have a low blood pressure (e.g. 60/90 mmHg). A rise to 'normal' levels (80/120 mmHg) may represent a significant elevation. Regular monitoring of blood pressure is essential as changes can occur quickly; monitor blood pressure every 5 minutes until blood pressure control is achieved.

Autonomic dysreflexia is considered a *medical emergency* and nurses need to ensure that the patient has medication prescribed, such as an antihypertensive (e.g. nifedipine), should this condition occur. Administer the prescribed medication and monitor the patient's blood pressure: if there is no response then call the crash team. Box 4.2 shows the treatment of autonomic dysreflexia in more detail.

NOTE: autonomic dysreflexia can usually be easily remedied by the removal of the cause of the painful stimuli, use of local anaesthetic and/or use of a vasodilator.

Box 4.2 Manifestations, causes and treatment for autonomic dysreflexia

Manifestations:

- Severe hypertension
- Bradycardia
- 'Pounding' headache
- Flushed or 'blotchy' skin above the level of lesion
- Pallor below the level of lesion
- Profuse sweating above the level of lesion
- Shortness of breath

Common causes:

- Any painful or noxious stimuli below the level of injury
- Distended bladder (usually due to catheter blockage or another form of bladder outlet obstruction)
- Distended bowel (usually due to a full rectum, constipation, or impaction)
- Skin problems/ingrowing toenail
- Fracture below the level of lesion
- Labour/childbirth
- Ejaculation (Glickman and Kamm 1996, Wiesel and Bell 2004)

Actions to take:

- Sit the patient up (where possible) to induce an element of postural hypotension.
- Ensure there is adequate urinary drainage (change the catheter if necessary, do not give a bladder washout/instillation).
- Empty the rectum by digital removal of faeces (local anaesthetic gel should be used).
- Blood pressure should be treated until the cause is found and eliminated (administer a proprietary vasodilator, e.g. nifedipine, as prescribed).
- If unable to locate cause, or symptoms persist, get help immediately.

THE PROCEDURES: STEP BY STEP

Procedural Steps for Digital Rectal Examination

Consider the circumstances when extra care is required, and also the exclusions and contra-indications. Before undertaking DRE abnormalities of the perineal and perianal area should be observed, looking for rectal prolapse, haemorrhoids, anal skin tags, wounds, dressings, discharge, anal lesions, gaping anus, skin condition, bleeding, faecal matter, infestation and foreign bodies.

Equipment required
Disposable latex-free gloves
Incontinence sheet/pad
Wipes
Lubricant (e.g. KY jelly)
Waste bag
Plastic apron

Intervention	Rationale
1 Check with patient and hospital notes for any contra-indications.	To minimise risk of potential problems
2 Explain the procedure and obtain verbal consent.	To reduce anxiety and gain consent
3 Ensure the procedure is carried out in the privacy of a cubicle or curtained area*.	To maintain patient's privacy and dignity
4 Wash hands with soap and water and put on apron and double gloves.	Prevent potential contact with body fluids and minimise the risk of cross-infection
5 Position the patient on their left side with their back next to the edge of the bed, and their knees flexed. Place an absorbent pad under the patient and cover the patient with a sheet.	Positioning allows ease of entry into the rectum following the natural curve of the colon
6 Examine the perianal area for any abnormalities before proceeding.	To ensure that it is safe to proceed
7 Reassure the patient throughout the procedure.	To avoid unnecessary stress or embarrassment and ensure continued consent
8 Lubricate gloved index finger and insert gently into the rectum. Note: nurses' nails must be kept short.	To minimise patient discomfort and avoid anal mucosal trauma

(continued)

Intervention	Rationale
9 Assess for the presence of faecal matter using the Bristol Stool Chart (see Figure 4.2).	To check for the presence of faecal matter and to establish the consistency of the stool
10 Slowly withdraw finger from patient's rectum when finished. Check for presence of faeces or blood on glove.	To minimise patient discomfort
11 Remove top glove and dispose of in clinical waste bag.	To minimise risk of cross-infection
12 Wipe residual lubricating gel from anal area.	To ensure the patient's comfort and avoid anal excoriation
13 Dispose of gloves, apron and equipment into a yellow bag and wash hands.	To prevent cross-infection
14 Ensure patient is comfortable and observe for any adverse reactions.	To and minimise embarrassment and note adverse reactions
15 Record findings in nursing documentation and communicate findings with medical team if appropriate; consistency, volume, date and time should all be recorded appropriately.	To ensure correct care and continuity of care

*Where available and appropriate DRE should be performed in the patient's side room to protect the privacy and dignity of the patient, and protect other patients from potential malodour.

Procedural Steps for Administration of Enemas and Suppositories

Consider the circumstances when extra care is required, and also the exclusions and contra-indications. Before inserting enemas or suppositories, abnormalities of the perineal and perianal area should be observed as per DRE. Special precautions also need to be assessed: recent colorectal surgery, malignancy (or other pathology) of the perianal region and low platelet count.

Equipment required
Disposable latex-free gloves
Incontinence sheet/pad
Wipes
Lubricant (e.g. KY jelly)
Waste bag
Plastic apron
Suppository or enema, prescribed by medic or nurse prescriber

Intervention	Rationale
1 Obtain verbal consent and document it.	To reduce anxiety and gain consent
2 Collect and prepare the equipment.	To ensure procedure is conducted in an efficient and timely manner, thus reducing anxiety
3 Take patient's pulse rate at rest prior to and during the procedure.	To record baseline pulse and monitor for changes
4 Take blood pressure in spinally injured patients prior to, during and at the end of the procedure.	To record baseline pulse and monitor for changes
5 Prepare the patient; assist with removing clothing from waist down, help in positioning patient on left lateral position, knees flexed, taking into consideration the normal line of the sigmoid colon.	Positioning allows ease of entry into the rectum following the natural curve of the colon
6 Protect bedding and mattress and wash hands with soap and water.	To maintain infection-control procedures and patient dignity
7 Observe the anal area and put on gloves and apron.	To ensure that it is safe to proceed; to prevent potential contact with body fluids and minimise the risk of cross-infection
8 Lubricate the gloved index finger; inform the patient that you are about to perform the procedure.	To minimise patient discomfort and avoid anal mucosal trauma
9 Gain patient co-operation by asking the patient to relax prior to insertion of index or middle finger.	To avoid unnecessary stress or embarrassment and ensure continued consent

(continued)

Intervention	Rationale
10 Insert the gloved finger into the anus slowly and on into the rectum.	To minimise patient discomfort and avoid anal mucosal trauma
11 Assess for faecal matter, document the amount and consistency, using the Bristol Stool Chart (see Figure 4.2). Assess the need for medication.	To establish rectal loading and the consistency of the stool
12 Lubricate the blunt end of the suppository or the tube tip of the enema (after cap has been removed); inform the patient that you are about to perform the procedure, then insert the suppository/enema via the anus into the rectum.	Inserting the suppository blunt end first allows the anal sphincter to assist with insertion (Abd-El-Maeboud et al. 1991).
13 Clean anal area; remove gel by wiping residual from area to ensure that it does not cause irritation or soreness.	To maintain cleanliness; to leave patient comfortable
14 Dispose of equipment as per local policy.	To prevent cross-infection
15 Help patient to get up and dressed and into a comfortable position; offer toileting facilities as appropriate.	To maintain dignity and to minimise embarrassment
16 Document procedure fully on completion.	To establish effectiveness of procedure; to ensure continuity of care

Procedural Steps for Digital Removal of Faeces

Consider the circumstances when extra care is required, and also the exclusions and contra-indications. Before undertaking DRF, abnormalities of the perineal and perianal area should be observed, as for DRE. When undertaking this procedure, the following observations and risk factors should be considered and documented, and medical assistance/advice should be sought:

- pulse at rest prior to procedure to obtain a baseline reading,
- pulse during procedure,
- blood pressure in spinal injury patients prior to, during and at the end of the procedure,
- signs and symptoms of autonomic dysreflexia (headache, flushing, sweating, hypertension),
- distress, pain, discomfort,
- bleeding,
- patient collapse.

Equipment required
Disposable latex-free gloves
Incontinence sheet/pad
Plastic apron
Wipes
Lubricant (e.g. KY jelly)
Soap and water
Clinical waste bag
Stethoscope
Sphygmomanometer
Bed pan/other suitable receptacle for waste

NOTE: This is a two-person procedure to ensure accurate and timely monitoring of observations during the procedure. Whereas a blood pressure monitor maybe useful in monitoring situations, in this instance manual pulse and blood pressure should be recorded to note rate, rhythm and amplitude.

Intervention	Rationale
1 Check with patient and hospital notes for any contra-indications.	To minimise risk of potential problems
2 Explain the procedure and obtain verbal consent.	To reduce anxiety and gain consent
3 Ensure procedure is carried out in the privacy of a cubicle or curtained area*.	To maintain patient's privacy and dignity
4 Take the patient's pulse rate at rest prior to the procedure.	To record baseline pulse and monitor for changes
5 Take the baseline blood pressure in all spinal injury patients.	To record baseline blood pressure and monitor for any changes

(continued)

Intervention	Rationale
6 Wash hands with soap and water and put on apron and double gloves.	Prevent potential contact with body fluids and minimise the risk of cross-infection
7 Position the patient on their left side with their back next to the edge of the bed, and their knees flexed. Place an absorbent pad under the patient and cover the patient with a sheet.	Positioning allows ease of entry into the rectum following the natural curve of the colon
8 Examine the perianal area for any abnormalities before proceeding.	To ensure that it is safe to proceed
9 For patients receiving this treatment on a regular basis use lubricating gel on the gloved index finger.	To minimise patient discomfort and avoid anal mucosal trauma
10 As an acute procedure, a local anaesthetic gel may be applied topically to the anal area. Wait for 5 minutes before proceeding. • Do not apply if anal mucosa is damaged. • Check for contra-indications.	To make the patient as comfortable and pain free as possible To ensure the anaesthetic gel has time to have the required effect
11 Reassure the patient throughout the procedure.	To avoid unnecessary stress or embarrassment and ensure continued consent
12 Insert lubricated gloved index finger into the rectum.	To minimise patient discomfort and avoid anal mucosal trauma
13 Assess for the presence of faecal matter using the Bristol Stool Chart (see Figure 4.2).	To establish rectal loading and the consistency of the stool
14 In type 1 stool (see Bristol Stool Chart) remove a lump at a time until the rectum is empty.	To minimise discomfort and facilitate easier removal of stool
15 In type 2 stool, push finger into the middle of the faecal mass and split it. Remove small sections of faeces at a time into appropriate receptacle.	To minimise discomfort and facilitate easier removal of stool
16 Do not overstretch sphincter by using a hooked finger to remove large pieces of stool.	To avoid trauma to the rectal mucosa and sphincter

Intervention	Rationale
17 If top glove becomes very soiled, remove and replace with a new top glove.	To avoid excessive soiling of patient's skin; to maintain cleanliness
18 Lubricate gloved finger with each change of top glove. Use extra lubrication as required.	To facilitate easier insertion and minimise friction and discomfort
19 If faecal mass is too hard, larger than 4 cm across, or you are unable to break it up, *stop* and refer to medical team.	To minimise risk of autonomic dysreflexia
20 If patient becomes distressed, check the pulse again and check against the baseline reading; *stop* if pulse rate has dropped, patient is distressed or if there is pain or bleeding in anal area. Check blood pressure for patients with spinal injury.	To monitor condition of patient and stop if necessary
21 When rectum is empty, remove top glove and clean and dry patient's perianal area.	To maintain cleanliness; to leave patient comfortable
22 Ensure skin is clean and dry. Observe skin on completion of procedure.	To monitor skin condition
23 Dispose of gloves, apron and equipment into a yellow bag and wash hands.	To prevent cross-infection
24 Ensure patient is comfortable and check pulse (and blood pressure for patients with spinal cord injury).	To observe for any adverse reactions
25 Record bowel results in nursing documentation and communicate results with patient/carer and medical team if appropriate. Consistency, volume, date and time should all be recorded appropriately. Report any abnormal findings immediately	To establish effectiveness of procedure; to ensure continuity of care

*Where available and appropriate DRF should be performed in the patient's side room or assisted bathroom to protect the privacy and dignity of the patient, and protect other patients from potential malodour.

Procedural Steps for Digital Rectal Stimulation

Consider the circumstances when extra care is required, and also the exclusions and contra-indications. Before undertaking DRS abnormalities of the perineal and perianal area should be observed, as per DRE. The following observations and risk factors should be considered and documented, and medical advice sought:

- pulse and blood pressure should be recorded before, during and after the procedure,
- signs and symptoms of autonomic dysreflexia in spinally injured patients,
- distress, pain, discomfort,
- patient collapse.

Equipment required
Disposable latex-free gloves
Incontinence sheet/pad
Plastic apron
Wipes
Lubricant (e.g. KY jelly)
Soap and water
Waste bag

Intervention	Rationale
1 Check with patient and hospital notes for any contra-indications.	To minimise risk of potential problems
2 Explain the procedure and obtain verbal consent.	To reduce anxiety and gain consent
3 Ensure procedure is carried out in the privacy of a cubicle or curtained area*.	To maintain patient's privacy and dignity
4 Wash hands with soap and water and put on apron and double gloves.	Prevent potential contact with body fluids and minimise the risk of cross-infection
5 Position the patient on their left side with their back next to the edge of the bed, and their knees flexed. Place an absorbent pad under the patient and cover the patient with a sheet.	Positioning allows ease of entry into the rectum following the natural curve of the colon
6 Examine the perianal area for any abnormalities before proceeding.	To ensure that it is safe to proceed

Intervention	Rationale
7 Reassure the patient throughout the procedure.	To avoid unnecessary stress or embarrassment and ensure continued consent
8 Lubricate gloved index finger and insert to the second joint of finger only.	To minimise patient discomfort and avoid anal mucosal trauma
9 Gently rotate the finger in a clockwise motion for 15–20 seconds or until internal sphincter relaxes. Note: circular motion originates from the wrist, not the finger.	To trigger reflex relaxation of internal sphincter and promote emptying of the rectum; the pad of the finger to the first joint stimulates reflex relaxation
10 Do not stimulate for more than 1 minute.	To prevent damage to anal sphincter
11 Stop if severe spasms of the anal sphincter occur, or if patient shows signs of autonomic dysreflexia.	Patient safety
12 Remove finger to allow faeces to pass.	To allow evacuation to take place
13 Stimulation cycle can be repeated up to three times.	To facilitate complete evacuation
14 Check rectum for presence of faeces. Proceed to manual evacuation if faeces present, but no faeces have been passed.	To ensure complete evacuation
15 Remove top glove and clean patient's perianal area with soap and water.	Reduces risk of cross-infection and ensures patient comfort
16 Ensure anal area is clean and dry. Observe skin on completion of procedure.	To prevent infection, contamination and excoriation of perianal area
17 Dispose of gloves, apron and equipment into a yellow bag and wash hands with soap and water.	To prevent cross-infection
18 Ensure patient is comfortable and observe for any adverse reactions.	To and minimise embarrassment and note adverse reactions
19 Record bowel results in nursing documentation and communicate results with patient/carer and medical team if appropriate. Consistency, volume, date and time should all be recorded appropriately.	To establish effectiveness of procedure; to ensure continuity of care

*Where available and appropriate DRS should be performed in the patient's side room or assisted bathroom to protect the privacy and dignity of the patient, and protect other patients from potential malodour.

TEST YOUR KNOWLEDGE

1 Name two functions of the bowel.
2 What is the stool assessment chart called?
3 What is DRE?
4 What does ADR stand for?
5 Name four trigger factors for ADR.
6 What is the purpose of digital rectal stimulation?

KEY POINTS

- Anatomy and physiology of the digestive system.
- The Bristol Stool Chart.
- Medications used in bowel dysfunction.
- Risk assessment.
- Performing a digital rectal examination.
- Digital removal of faeces.
- Digital rectal stimulation.
- Causes and treatment of autonomic dysreflexia.

Chapter 5

TRACHEOSTOMY CARE

Clinical Skills for Nurses, First Edition. Claire Boyd
© 2013 John Wiley & Sons, Ltd. Published 2013 by John Wiley & Sons Ltd.

LEARNING OUTCOMES

By the end of this chapter you will have an understanding of the theory and practice of performing the clinical skill of tracheostomy care.

A tracheostomy is an opening made in the anterior wall of the trachea to facilitate breathing (Figure 5.1) and may be performed to:

- bypass an upper airway obstruction, such as a tumour, cogenital abnormality or trauma, including head and neck or maxillofacial surgery;
- assist prolonged ventilation due to a neuromuscular disorder, coma or respiratory failure.

Before we start, you may want to reacquaint yourself with some of the terminology we used in relation to respiration in Chapter 1, such as hypoxia and hypercapnia.

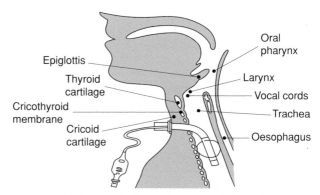

Figure 5.1 Placement of a tracheostomy tube in the trachea. Permission to reproduce this image is granted by North Bristol NHS Trust and University Hospitals Bristol NHS Foundation Trust

ANATOMY AND PHYSIOLOGY

Table 5.1 The upper airway

Nose	Air is drawn into the nasal cavity and is warmed and humidified so that it reaches the core temperature and saturation in the lungs. The inspired air is also cleaned and filtered to make it free of contaminants.
Pharynx	Three parts: nasopharynx, oropharynx and laryngopharynx
Epiglottis	This large piece of cartilage moves down and forms a lid over the airway when swallowing, so that food enters the oesophagus only, and not the larynx. Usually, if anything other than air enters the larynx the cough reflex is triggered to expel the foreign matter.
Larynx	Contains the vocal cords (which have an avascular, pearly white appearance): air passes over the vocal cords to make the sounds used in speech and other vocalisations.

The effect of by-passing the upper airway (Table 5.1) when a patient has a tracheostomy *in situ* is that the inspired air is not warmed, humidified or filtered. The lower respiratory system is outlined in Table 5.2.

Table 5.2 The lower respiratory system

Trachea	Continuation of the larynx: approximately 11.5 cm in length and 2.5 cm in diameter. It starts at the lower border of the cricoid cartilage (the only complete circle of cartilage) and ends at the bifurcating level of the bronchus. The lumen is kept open by incomplete cartilaginous rings. The *thyroid gland* lies lateral to the trachea. The gland is attached to the trachea by dense connective tissues.
Carina	Where the trachea divides into two main bronchi. Can be damaged by poor suctioning technique.
Right and left bronchus, and bronchioles and alveoli	Alveoli are made up of approximately 300 million cells, which possess thin walls to allow gaseous exchange. Alveoli contain oxygen, but during disease may become porous and blood-, bacteria- and pus-filled; this may create a crackling sound during inspiration and/or expiration.
The lungs	The right lung consists of three lobes. The left lung consists of two lobes (due to the heart).

The mucociliary transport system is the lining that extends from the nasopharynx to the respiratory bronchioles. This is the only fully functional mechanical barrier against inhaled or aspirated contaminants for patients with tracheostomies. It consists of three layers:

1 ciliated epithelial cells,
2 cilia and aqueous layer,
3 mucus layer.

Contaminants are moved by the cilia as they become trapped in the mucus layer. Cilia have hooked ends and beat with a wavelike movement. This mucus layer must be moist and not too thick, otherwise the contaminants will be too difficult to move; therefore they must have **humidification**. Without humidification, oxygen causes moisture and heat loss, resulting in thick secretions and what we call 'plugging'.

The lungs' optimal temperature is 37°C. This equates to a humidity of 44 mg/L (100%).

If the temperature is only 36°C, then the humidity is 42 mg/L. At 35°C the humidity is 40 mg/L, and at 30°C it is 30 mg/L.

If the humidity is anything less than saturated, the cilia are unable to beat and the gel layer loses moisture. If the temperature of the lungs is lower than the core temperature, the cilia beat less frequently and the relative humidity of the inspired air will be lost, resulting in pooling of mucus in the airway. If less-than-optimal humidification continues, then cell damage occurs and the cilia die. Remember that piped oxygen is colder in the winter, and therefore you may need to raise the temperature slightly.

TRACHEOSTOMY TUBES

There are many different types of tracheostomy tube, such as the following.

Cuffed Tracheostomy Tube

The advantage of this design (see Figure 5.2) is that when the cuff is inflated it prevents gas from escaping around the tube, enabling assisted ventilation and respiratory support.

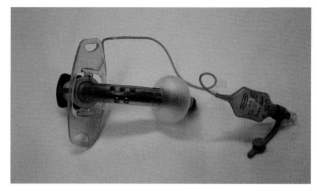

Figure 5.2 A cuffed tracheostomy tube

It also reduces the risk of large-volume aspiration of pharyngeal and gastric secretions into the trachea and lungs, and nosocomial pneumonia. When the pilot balloon is deflated, the cuff is deflated. The cuff pressure is usually measured every 6 hours.

NOTE: a speaking valve must never be placed on a cuffed tracheostomy tube. The tracheostomy cuff is made of a soft plastic that when inflated exerts low pressure on the trachea wall.

Un-cuffed Fenestrated Tracheostomy Tube

The advantage of this design (see Figure 5.3) is that the tube has fenestrations (holes) in the shaft of the tube. These holes direct airflow to pass through the patient's nasal/oral pharynx as well as the tracheostomy during breathing. This facilitates weaning the patient off the tube.

NOTE: when suctioning is required an inner tube without fenestrations should be inserted prior to the procedure.

Adjustable-Flange Tracheostomy Tube

The advantage of this design is that patients with deep-set tracheas (for example, secondary to obesity, distorted anatomy due to oedema, or musculoskeletal deformity such as kyphoscoliosis) can have the tube adjusted to the desired length. These tubes are normally cuffed.

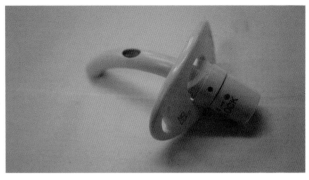

Figure 5.3 An un-cuffed tracheostomy tube

Cricothyroidotomy or Mini-Tracheostomy Tube

The advantage of this type of tube is that is can be inserted by non-surgeons for life-threatening airway obstruction in emergency situations. It can be used in patients experiencing sputum retention and requiring regular suctioning. Laryngeal function is preserved, including coughing, speaking and swallowing, and natural humidification is not disrupted.

Most tracheostomy tubes are changed every 28 days, or depending on the manufacturer's instructions, by experienced surgeons or staff.

Inner Cannula

Tracheostomy tubes may come as a one-piece tube or as a two-piece, meaning it has a inner cannula. An inner cannula:

- allows maintenance of tube patency,
- can be quickly removed if blocked,
- facilitates less frequent tracheostomy tube changes due to secretions being cleaned from the inner cannula, thus not building up on the tube itself.

An inner cannula reduces the diameter of the lumen of the tube, which may increase the patient's breathing workload. The inner cannula is usually cleaned every 6 hours and replaced every 7 days.

SUCTIONING TECHNIQUE

Patients require suctioning when they are unable to effectively clear their airway. Suctioning is required to remove secretions with minimal tissue damage and hypoxia (Box 5.1).

Box 5.1   Patient assessment to indicate suctioning

Signs/symptoms

Abnormal respiratory pattern
- **Increased respiratory rate**
- **Accessory muscle usage**
- **Increased work of breathing**

Changes in secretions
- **Increased quantity: infection,**
- **Increased tenacity: inadequate humidification**
- **Colour: infection, trauma (blood-stained)**

Persistent coughing

Change in skin colour
- **Cyanosis/clammy**

Visible or audible secretions

Anxiety/agitation

Note: patient assessment should include a full ABCDE assessment (see Chapter 10).

Extra consideration as to whether suction is appropriate should be given in the following circumstances:

- pulmonary oedema (use caution: consider the cause),
- hypoxia unless caused by secretions or a blocked tracheostomy tube,
- cardiovascular instability,
- uncontrolled clotting/INR (see Chapter 8),
- severe bronchospasm.

NOTE: seek guidance from a senior nurse, physiotherapist or doctor.

Equipment

Patients with a tracheostomy *must* have the following equipment for performing suction available at their bedside prior to arrival on the ward/unit:

- suction canister,
- suction tubing (change at least once a week or when heavily soiled: infection-control direction),
- suction catheters of correct size (see below for guidelines).
- Yankauer sucker for oral care (single-use only),
- gloves,
- aprons,
- eye protection,
- sterile water: change at least every 24 hours,
- small bowl with lid: change at least every 24 hours,
- oxygen, tubing and tracheostomy mask,
- clinical waste bag for disposal of clinical equipment.

Suction Catheter Size and Suction Pressure

Choosing a suction catheter of the right size (Table 5.3) is essential for safe and efficient suctioning. The external diameter of the suction catheter should not be greater than half of the internal diameter of the tracheostomy tube.

Table 5.3 Quick reference to catheter size

Tube inner diameter	Suction catheter size
6 mm	8–10
7 mm	10–12
8 mm	12–14
9 mm	14

The pressure of the suction should be at 60–150 mmHg when suction is applied. Greater pressures may cause atelectasis.

If secretions are very tenacious then an increase in the suction catheter size is recommended, rather than increasing the vacuum pressure above 150 mmHg.

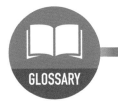

Atelectasis
Failure of part of the lung to expand due to immature cells lining the alveoli (i.e. in premature babies) or damage.

Procedure

1 Inform the patient of the procedure and gain informed consent.
2 Check suction is on and working and set to correct pressure.
3 Wash hands and apply apron and goggles.
4 If the existing cannula is fenestrated, change to a plain inner cannula.
5 Attach suction catheter to the suction tubing using a clean technique.
6 Place clean gloves on hands or place a second glove on your dominant hand if gloves are already worn. Do not touch anything other than the unsheathed catheter with the glove on the dominant hand.
7 Remove catheter from sheathing using a clean technique, aiming not to touch the end third of the catheter.
8 Maintain the patient's oxygen *in situ* wherever possible.
9 Gently insert the catheter into the tracheostomy tube without suction applied, until either a cough is stimulated or resistance of the carina is felt.
10 The catheter should be then withdrawn 0.5–1 cm before suction is applied.
11 Withdraw the catheter slowly with suction applied continuously. The catheter should not be rotated.
12 Reapply oxygen if required and observe and reassess patient. Allow the patient to recover before repeating the procedure if required.
13 Inspect the secretions prior to disposing of catheter and gloves and flush through suction tubing with sterile water. (Suction catheters are single-use only.)
14 Change inner cannula back to fenestrated if required.

15 Evaluate the effectiveness of suctioning and document and report as required.

NOTE: suctioning should last no longer than 10–15 seconds from insertion to removal of the catheter.

Complications of suctioning can be seen in Table 5.4.

Table 5.4 Complications of suctioning

Complication	Potential causes	Action
Hypoxia	Prolonged suctioning and by removing the oxygen given by the tracheostomy mask	Consider 'staging' suction episodes Pre-oxygenate Liaise with physiotherapist/medical staff
Mucosal trauma (e.g. blood-stained secretions)	Poor suction technique	Consider 'measured-depth' suctioning: use the measurements on a suction catheter to measure the depth of the carina. After this only insert subsequent catheters to 1 cm less than the depth of the carina. Gain expert advice.
Infection	Insertion of a contaminated suction catheter	Revise technique. Inform medical staff.
Anxiety	Stress and discomfort of being suctioned and enforced coughing	Reassure and explain necessity.
Pain	Poor technique and 'jabbing the carina' or pain at sites of surgery due to coughing	Revise technique. Gain medical opinion if pain continues.
Cardiac arrhythmias	Vaso–vagal response caused by tracheal stimulation by catheter, or severe hypoxia	Inform medical staff. Consider pre-oxygenation.
Raised intracranial pressure	Stimulation of trachea causing coughing	Stagger frequency of suctioning.
Secretions are not clearing easily	Lack of humidification/patient hydration	Consider reviewing humidification/patient hydration, or using saline nebulisers (consult physiotherapist/medical staff).

Complication	Potential causes	Action
Patient has pain that is limiting coughing	Pain	Review analgesia.
Patient has high levels of anxiety related to suction		Inform and reassure.
It is difficult to pass a suction catheter down the tracheostomy tube	Build-up of secretions in inner cannula. If secretions are absent, consider tracheal stenosis or granuloma: request an ear/nose/throat (ENT) review urgently.	Remove inner cannula for duration of suctioning only.

CUFF PRESSURE MONITORING

It is recommended that the cuffs of the tracheostomy tube are maintained at a pressure of 20–25 mmHg (unless instructions state otherwise). Lower pressures prevent optimal ventilation. Higher pressures can compress mucosal capillaries, which can lead to ischaemia and tracheal stenosis. The pressure should be checked every 6 hours with a designed for purpose pressure gauge.

PROCEDURE FOR CLEANING AND DRESSING THE TRACHEOSTOMY STOMA SITE

The stoma site should be clean and dry to minimise the risk of skin irritation and infection. Secretions collected above the tracheostomy tube cuff may ooze out of the surgical incision and stoma site, leading to skin maceration and excoriation. This increased moisture may act as a medium for bacterial growth and/or prevent the stoma site from healing.

The stoma site should be assessed at least once every 6 hours, for trauma, infection or inflammation. Findings should be recorded in the tracheostomy care plan and any problems should be reported as necessary to the senior nurse and/or the doctor.

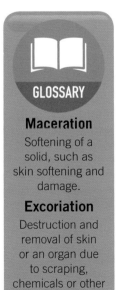

GLOSSARY

Maceration
Softening of a solid, such as skin softening and damage.

Excoriation
Destruction and removal of skin or an organ due to scraping, chemicals or other means.

If Velcro tapes are used, these will need to be assessed at least every 4 hours. This is due to the fact that when wet these tapes may stretch, allowing the tracheostomy tube to dislodge. A two-finger technique should be used to secure tube (see procedure, below).

The dressing and tapes may need to be changed more frequently (e.g. if they become soiled).

The cleaning and dressing of the tracheostomy stoma site is a two-person task to prevent dislodgement of the tracheostomy, and if required during an emergency situation.

Red, excoriated or exuding stomas should be swabbed and the doctor informed. Advice should be sought from the wound care team for the treatment of complicated wounds.

Ensure the patient has had adequate analgesia prior to the procedure, as patients may experience pain and discomfort during the dressing change.

Some tracheostomy tubes are secured with sutures and some may have stat/rescue sutures in place. These sutures require attention upon cleaning, as they are potential sites of infection.

Guidelines for Cleaning and Dressing the Tracheostomy Stoma Site

Action	Rationale
1 Ensure two people are available prior to undertaking the procedure.	By removing the tracheostomy tapes, the tracheostomy tube may dislodge. One practitioner therefore holds the tube in place while the other performs the procedure.
2 Check emergency equipment.	To ensure patient safety if the tracheostomy tube dislodges
3 Explain procedure to the patient and reassure them.	To ensure that the patient understands the procedure, co-operates and gives consent; to reduce patient anxiety
4 Check suction equipment.	To ensure patient safety if patient requires tracheal suctioning during procedure

Action	Rationale
5 Screen bed space.	To ensure patient privacy
6 Wash hands. Put on apron and gloves.	To reduce the risk of cross-infection
7 Position patient with neck slightly extended (if patient's medical condition allows).	To allow easier access to the stoma site and maintain optimum airway alignment
8 Put on goggles and perform tracheal suctioning, if required.	To reduce the risk of cross-infection from the patient's secretions
9 Wash hands. Don clean apron.	To prevent infection
10 Prepare dressing trolley using aseptic technique.	To ensure the technique is as clean as possible, and all equipment is easily accessible
11 Unfasten oxygen mask: assisting practitioner to hold in place over tracheostomy site while at the same time holding tracheostomy tube in place.	To ensure patient's oxygen requirements are maintained; to ensure tracheostomy tube is stabilised and to reduce the risk of dislodgement
12 Remove Velcro tape or ties and old dressing.	To facilitate replacing with new tape/ties and dressing and to reduce infection
13 Discard soiled Velcro tape/ties and dressing into clinical waste bag.	To reduce the risk of cross-infection (refer to waste management policy)
14 Assess tracheostomy stoma site for signs of trauma, infection, inflammation and/or maceration. Take a swab if any signs of infection.	To detect and treat stoma complications early to reduce the risk of deterioration of the stoma site
15 Clean gently around stoma site with 0.9% sodium chloride and gauze. Dry thoroughly.	To remove secretions and crusts; to reduce trauma to tracheostomy site (other cleaning agents may cause irritation to the tracheal mucosa and surrounding skin); to reduce the risk of infection
16 Apply Lyofoam (or similar) keyhole dressing, starting from below the stoma, placing dressing pink side uppermost.	To ensure the patient's comfort by minimising the risk of pressure, shearing and friction from the tracheostomy tube

(continued)

Action	Rationale
17 Secure in place with ties and tracheostomy foam tube holder or Velcro tracheostomy tape. The tape/ties should be tight enough to keep the tracheostomy tube securely in place but loose enough to allow two fingers to fit between the ties and neck. If using Velcro tape to secure, assess 4 hourly.	To promote patient comfort and reduce trauma from a migrating tracheostomy tube; to minimise the risk of reduced cerebral blood flow from the carotid arteries due to excessive external pressure; to assess Velcro tapes are not wet, which may cause stretching to the tapes and tracheostomy tube to become dislodged
18 Refasten oxygen mask and re-position patient for comfort.	To prevent the risk of hypoxia; to promote patient comfort
19 Dispose of all soiled equipment.	To prevent the risk of cross-infection
20 Record procedure and stoma site assessment in patient's notes and/or care plan. Report to doctor and refer to wound care team if further action is required.	To facilitate communication and evaluation: optimal care requires a multi-professional approach.

TEST YOUR KNOWLEDGE

There may have been some words used in this chapter that you have not come across before and not understood. Hopefully you looked these words up in a medical dictionary. What do the following words mean?

1 tenacious
2 bifurcating
3 kyphoscoliosis
4 INR

KEY POINTS

- Anatomy and physiology of the upper and lower airways.
- Tracheostomy tubes.
- Suctioning techniques and complications.
- Cleaning and dressing the tracheostomy stoma site.

Chapter 6
· · · · · · · · · · · · · · · · · · · ·
POINT-OF-CARE TRAINING

Clinical Skills for Nurses, First Edition. Claire Boyd
© 2013 John Wiley & Sons, Ltd. Published 2013 by John Wiley & Sons Ltd.

LEARNING OUTCOMES

By the end of this chapter you will have an understanding of the theory and practice of performing the clinical skill of point-of-care training: urinalysis, faecal occult blood testing and blood glucose monitoring.

Point-of-care training is when we conduct pathology testing at the 'point of care' – that is, in the clinical area – rather than sending the sample (e.g. blood, urine, faeces) in the first instance to the biochemistry laboratory to be tested. Some areas call this 'near-patient testing'.

NOTE: all of these tests require training and assessment prior to you being able to perform these procedures.

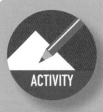

ACTIVITY

Activity 6.1

Before we get started let's test your knowledge of urine to see how much you know.
1   What is the pH value of healthy urine?
2   What might a low urine pH value indicate?
3   To what might a low urine pH indicate a predisposition?
4   What might a high urine pH value indicate?
5   What is the most common cause of a high urine pH reading?

URINALYSIS

There are many urine-testing sticks on the market (Figure 6.1): these are sometimes referred to as 'dip sticks' or reagent strips. The ones that we shall be looking at are called Combur 5 and Combur 7, manufactured by Roche, but the technique and overview is predominately

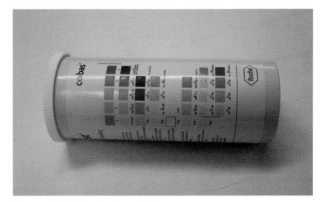

Figure 6.1 Urinalysis test strips

the same whichever testing kit you use. You will of course need to check the instructions given by the testing kit's manufacturer.

It should be remembered that all patient samples are a potential infection risk and health and safety procedures must be adhered to, including disposal of used materials.

The Combur 5 urine test strip is used to detect urine pH, and the presence of glucose, ketones, proteins and blood or haemoglobin in the urine sample. The Combur 7 urine test strip is used to detect the urine pH, plus glucose, ketones, leucocytes, nitrite, protein and blood. Figure 6.1 shows these test strips.

To perform the test, you will require a test strip kit, your fob watch for timing, an apron and gloves, and a paper hand towel or two. You will also require a collection container. There are a few prerequisites to performing this test, one is to check that the test strips have been stored correctly with the cap intact, out of direct sunlight and away from extremes of temperature. The other is that the person conducting this test is not colour blind.

The Sample

The sample must be collected in an uncontaminated container: this means something that has not been cleaned with disinfectant. Foil or paper-mache containers are ideal for this type of sample collection and the patient's details should be written on the container. The best urine to collect for this test is an early morning urine (EMU) sample, collected midstream (MSU). Your patient may not know what this means, so you may need to explain it to them as well as asking them to clean the genital area before providing the sample. Children and immobile patients may need assistance with sample collection.

For detection of diabetes, a sample collected roughly 2 hours after a meal is preferred. A urine sample should not be tested more than 2 hours after it has been produced, or contain blood, faeces or cream, etc., as this will contaminate the sample and the test will have to be repeated. Once a sample has been obtained, and mixed well, the assessment begins: First we inspect the colour and smell.

The Test

1 Wash and dry your hands and put on gloves and apron. Ensure you have a good light source under which to conduct this test.
2 Check the expiry date of the strips on the container and that the cap still contains loose desiccant (indicating that the test strips have not got damp). If the desiccant in the cap is not loose (i.e. it is in one large clump) it may be indicative that dampness has contaminated the test strips.
3 Remove a test strip from the container. Hold the white end of the test strip and inspect the test pads. The pads should look slightly lighter than the left-hand lines of pads on the colour chart on the strip container.
4 Immerse the pads in the urine sample for no longer than 1 second.
5 Remove the test strip from the urine by dragging the reverse side of the test strip over the edge of the sample container to remove the excess urine.
6 Place the test strip face up on a paper towel (check that the towel does not contain high levels of starch).
7 Wait for exactly 60 seconds.

8 Read the test strip against the colour chart on the test strip container immediately after the 60 seconds are up. The colour will continue to develop: if the time has gone beyond 120 seconds then discard the strip and repeat the test.

9 When reading the strip, make sure that it is orientated correctly and that the pads line up with the correct portions of the colour chart. The pad nearest the holding strip should be in line with the pH chart.

10 Results: for each pad select the colour block on the chart that *most closely matches the pad* (Figure 6.2).

Record all the parameters measured: the pH and results and numbers from each of the pads. The results from a test shown in Figure 6.3 would need to be recorded and reported. They show:

pH 5
+3 Glucose
+2 Ketones
+1 Leucocytes
Negative Nitrite
+ 2 Protein
Negative Blood

If the patient's results are not consistent with their condition, retest with a freshly collected sample. Table 6.1 highlights the issues to consider when checking a urinalysis result.

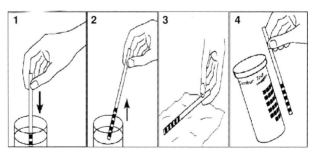

Figure 6.2 Urinalysis procedure. Permission to reproduce this image is granted by North Bristol NHS Trust and University Hospitals Bristol NHS Foundation Trust

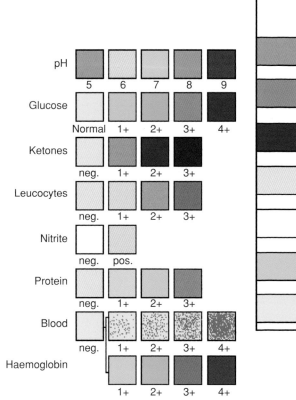

Figure 6.3 Urinalysis results. Permission to reproduce this image is granted by North Bristol NHS Trust and University Hospitals Bristol NHS Foundation Trust

Table 6.1 Issues to consider when checking urinalysis results

Diet, medication or disease may alter the colour or smell of the urine. Some drugs, foods or infections can colour the urine, e.g. co-danthramer, beetroot, red cells (red), methylene blue (green), rifampicin (red-orange), nitrofurantoin, bilirubin (deep yellow), L-dopa, metronidazole (red brown) and *Pseudomonas* infection (blue-green). Foul-smelling or cloudy urine may indicate infection. Stale-smelling (ammoniacal) urine may be due to stagnation.	The pH will be falsely elevated if the urine has been left longer than 2 hours before the test is performed.

If the patient is not clean, the urine may be contaminated and an incorrect result reported.	The protein may be falsely positive if the pH is below 5 and falsely negative if the pH is above 9.
Blood may be present due to menstruation. Allow 2 days before and 2 days after menstruation.	Vegetarians often have a pH that is above 9.
The test strips should only be used on urine samples, and not any other type of fluid (pleural fluids, knee fluids, cerebral spinal fluid, etc.).	Ketones can be present after a long fast. Ignore any red colour on the pad. High doses of salicylate will reduce the colour.
The blood/haemoglobin pad colour may be reduced by excess proteins or by an infected urine sample.	If glucose is positive for a person who has *not* been diagnosed with diabetes, further investigation is required.

What does it all mean?

Depending on the test kit you are using, urinalysis can be used to show early signs and symptoms of many diseases, such as:

- liver disease,
- renal disease,
- diabetes mellitus,
- hypertension,
- pre-eclampsia,
- biliary disease,
- renal stones,
- malignant tumours.

Glucose is not normally present in urine and its presence may indicate that renal absorption is abnormal, or that the patient has raised blood glucose levels.

Ketones in the urine may indicate uncontrolled diabetes or anorexia.

Protein in the urine may indicate hypertension, pre-eclampsia, glomerulonephritis, infection or diabetes.

Blood in the urine may indicate infection, renal stones, injury to the renal tract or kidneys, or malignancy.

Nitrite may be indicative of infection. The sample of urine for this test should be obtained from urine passed 4 hours after the last voiding, or be an early morning sample.

Bilirubin in the urine may indicate hepatic disease.

FAECAL OCCULT BLOOD TEST

As with urine testing there are many different test kits on the market for this test and the one we shall be looking at is the Hema-screen test kit (made by Immunostics). The test is designed to detect the presence of abnormal amounts of blood in the faeces.

Faecal *occult* blood testing just means that the blood may not be apparent to the naked eye: hence the use of chemical slides to detect the 'hidden' blood.

This test is useful in the assessment of patients with gastrointestinal symptoms with anaemia and is used in screening asymptomatic patients for colorectal cancer.

To perform the test, you will require a test kit (containing the test slides, developer and applicator), your fob watch, apron, gloves, collection container for the sample and some paper towels. Figure 6.4 shows the test slide.

The test kit should have been stored correctly, away from extremes of humidity. Again, as with urine testing the person conducting the test should not be colour blind.

The sample should be fresh and collected in a container that has not be cleaned with disinfectant: foil or paper-mache containers are ideal. Whichever type of container is used, it must have the patient's details clearly written on. We need to inform our patient that the sample must be free from urine or any other potential contaminants, with the genitals cleaned prior to sample collection. Some patients may require assistance with the sample collection.

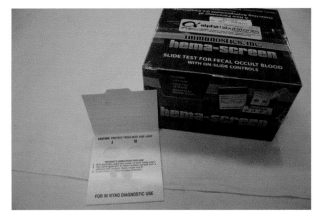

Figure 6.4 Faecal occult blood testing slide

This test is invalid in female patients for 3 days before and after menstruation (GPs may suggest just 2 days if this test is performed at home).

Dietary Preparation

Dietary preparation is important to uncover colorectal carcinoma. The patient requires dietary restrictions for 3 days, as certain foods can give incorrect recordings (false positives and false negatives). This requires the patient avoiding:

- high fibre,
- red meat,
- raw vegetables,
- raw fruit,
- horseradish,
- parsnips,
- turnips,
- melon,
- broccoli,
- excess vitamin C (above 0.5 g/day),
- excess iron (above 1 g/day).

It is usual for asymptomatic patients to require three individual collections over a 3-day period.

The Test

1 Wash and dry your hands and put on apron and gloves.

2 Check the expiry date on the test slide and developer bottle.

3 Remove the test slide from the kit and write the patient's details on the front section of the slide.

4 Open the flap of the slide and check that the test areas are cream-coloured. If they have a bluish tint do not use the slide.

5 Use one end of your applicator stick and smear a pea-sized sample of faeces over oval I.

6 Use the other end of the applicator stick to take a second pea-sized sample of faeces from a different area of the sample and smear this over oval II.

7 Now close the front flap and turn the slide over and wait for a minimum of 2 minutes or a maximum of 14 days for the sample to react with the slide.

8 Open the back flap of the slide and apply two drops of the developer to each oval. Time for exactly 60 seconds.

9 After 60 seconds read the results from the ovals.

10 Place one drop of developer onto the control area. For the test to be valid the POS (positive) areas must change to blue and the NEG (negative) areas must remain clear. If the control area does not do this, then repeat the test with a fresh slide.

11 A positive result is when there is any trace of blue colouring in either of the test areas. A negative result is when there is no blue colouring in either test area. Document and report your results. Figure 6.5 shows examples of positive and negative results.

Sources of Blood in the Faeces

- *Normal blood loss*: normal faecal blood loss is about 1–2 mL/day. The Hema-screen test detects blood amounts of 3–6 mL/day.
- *Clinical conditions*: bowel and colon disease, tumours, ulcers (both stomach and intestines) and haemorrhoids.

(a)

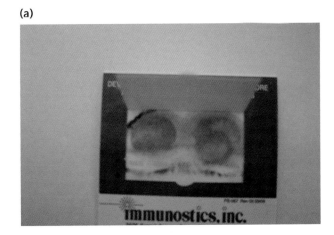

(b)

Figure 6.5 Faecal occult blood test results. **(a)** Blue present, meaning a positive result. **(b)** No blue present, which is a negative result

- *Medication*: aspirin, indomethacin, corticosteroids, reserpine, phenylbutazone, etc.
- *Artefactual*: menstrual bleeding, dental work, blood from tester's hands.

Table 6.2 highlights the issues to be considered when checking blood in the faeces.

Table 6.2 Issues to consider when checking blood in the faeces

If the patient is not clean, the sample may be contaminated and an incorrect result reported.	Blood may be present due to menstruation. Allow 3 days before and 3 days after menstruation before faecal occult blood testing (GPs may suggest just 2 days if this test is performed at home).
Colorectal cancers can bleed intermittently and may require a change of diet and collections on three separate days to detect bleeding.	False positives may occur if large amounts of raw fruit, vegetables, fibre, horseradish, parsnips, turnips, melon, broccoli or red meat are present in the diet.
Excessive vitamin C intake can give falsely negative results.	Iron-containing preparations may cause false-positive results to be seen, although a normal therapeutic dose (3 × 65 mg/day) should not interfere with the results. Iron may also turn the faeces black, thus masking the positive blue colour.
The test slides should only be used on faecal samples, not any other type of fluid (pleural fluids, knee fluids, cerebral spinal fluid, etc.).	The use of rectal preparations may interfere with the testing process.

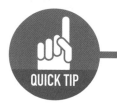

QUICK TIP

The recommended daily allowance for vitamin C varies. In the UK is 60 mg per day, although some countries, such as the USA, recommendations are much higher than this (3000 mg!).

If the test results are inconsistent with the patient's condition, retest with a fresh sample.

As with the urinalysis testing, it should be remembered that all patient samples are a potential infection risk and health and safety procedures must be adhered to, including disposal of used materials. One other consideration for the Hema-screen test is that the developer is flammable and should be kept well away from potential ignition sources.

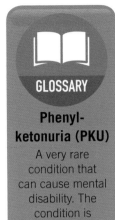

Phenyl-ketonuria (PKU)

A very rare condition that can cause mental disability. The condition is treatable once diagnosed.

BLOOD LANCING

Blood lancing is performed to obtain capillary blood samples. One reason to do it is to obtain a drop of blood to put on a slide for testing in a blood glucose monitor. This is the only way we can perform a blood glucose monitoring test.

Blood lancing is also performed to obtain blood samples during a 'heel-prick test' on babies. This test can identify a range of conditions, such as sickle cell disease, cystic fibrosis, phenylketonuria (PKU) and congenital hypothyroidism.

The device we shall be looking at for this procedure is the Unistik blood lancet (manufactured by Owen Mumford). There are four different types of Unistik lancets (Table 6.3), depending on gauge and patient.

Table 6.3 Unistik lancets

Comfort	Gauge: 28 G Depth: 1.8 mm To be used for blood glucose analysis
Neonatal	Gauge: 18 G Depth: 1.8 mm To be used for neonatal screening only
Normal	Gauge: 23 G Depth: 1.8 mm
Extra	Gauge: 21 G Depth: 2.0 mm To be used for haemoglobinometers only

The Test

1 Wash and dry your hands and put on gloves and apron.
2 Clean the sampling site with soap and warm water. Do not use alcohol wipes, as this cools the site and hardens the skin over time. Dry the collection site thoroughly.
3 Ensure that there is a good blood supply to the sampling site. This can be achieved by positioning

the limb so that it is hanging down or by warming the sample site, or by getting the patient to exercise the limb.

4 Select the correct type of Unistik 3 lancet.
5 Rotate the cap until it comes free. This usually takes two or three rotations.
6 Remove the cap and discard it.
7 Position the Unistik 3 lancet so that it is within the correct sampling zones; that is, on the upper outer aspects of the fingers or on a baby's outer heel. Press down firmly.
8 Press the release button on the lancet.
9 After blood collection, use gauze and gentle pressure until the blood flow stops.

Blood sampling sites are the upper outer aspects of the fingers. Try to avoid the thumb and index finger. If repeat sampling is required, it is important to rotate the sampling site.

The sampling area for a baby is on the outer aspects of the side heel. Migration from this sampling zone on baby's heel will cause calcification of the heel and long-term problems with mobility for the baby.

The type of lancet used for blood lancing is designed to be less painful when lancing. You will notice that the end platform of the lancet has a circle of raised bumps (Figure 6.6). These activate the C nerve fibres in the skin. These fibres can gate the pain transmitted by the $A\alpha$ and $A\beta$ nerve fibres, which should reduce the pain felt by the patient.

Table 6.4 highlights issues to consider when using Unistik.

Table 6.4 Issues to consider when using Unistik

Make sure that you use the correct version of the Unistik 3.	Always stay within the correct blood collection zones.

The lancet should be discarded into the nearest sharps container.

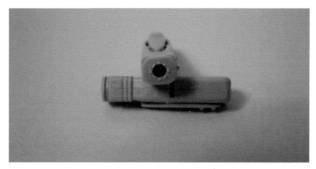

Figure 6.6 Raised circle of bumps on a blood lancet

BLOOD GLUCOSE TESTING

There are many different devices on the market to monitor a patient's blood glucose level. This section will look at the principles of blood glucose monitoring and will not focus on using any specific machine. You will of course need to be trained for the device your clinical area presently uses. These devices can be held in the hand or placed on large station ports.

The patient will first require to have one of their digits lanced, to obtain the blood sample. Blood glucose monitoring is usually conducted on all patients during routine admission and on patients with diabetes.

Blood Glucose Levels

The blood glucose and 'blood sugar levels' are synonymous terms used to express the amount of glucose present in the blood, known as the plasma glucose level. Normal blood glucose levels vary throughout the day but tend to remain between 4 and 8 mmol/L, being lowest in the early morning and higher after meals. Ideal values may be:

- 4–7 mmol/L before meals,
- less than 10 mmol/L 90 minutes after a meal,
- around 8 mmol/L at bedtime.

However, it should always be remembered that we are individuals and our 'norm' may vary from the 'ideal'. Also, in cardiopulmonary resuscitation a blood glucose reading of 4–10 mmol/L is often the acceptable range.

People with diabetes may have more fluctuations in their blood glucose levels and may need to be monitored more closely. Table 6.5 shows the different types of diabetes.

Table 6.5 Different types of diabetes

Type of diabetes	May also be known as	Information
Type 1 diabetes	Insulin-dependent diabetes mellitus (IDDM)	The body is unable to produce insulin. Usually starts in childhood or young adulthood. Treated with dietary control and insulin injections. Regular physical activity is recommended.
Type 2 diabetes	Non-insulin-dependent diabetes mellitus (NIDDM)	The body does not produce enough insulin or this insulin does not work properly (insulin resistance). Tends to affect people as they get older, usually appearing after the age of 40, but it is increasingly being seen in younger, overweight and obese people. Treated with diet and physical activity or by diet, physical activity and oral medication. May require insulin therapy as disease progresses.

Normal Blood Sugar Control: the Science Bit

The glucose that we ingest from sweet and starchy foods gets turned into energy. Insulin is a hormone manufactured by the pancreas and it regulates the amount of glucose in the blood. When levels of glucose in the body rise, such as just after eating a meal, the pancreas is triggered to release insulin, which then starts to stimulate the cells in the body to absorb the glucose. Without insulin the glucose levels in the blood would just keep rising and cells in the body would be unable to utilise it for energy, resulting in extreme tiredness, as often experienced by those with untreated diabetes. Insulin also stimulates the liver to absorb some of the glucose and store any that is left over. The pancreas also manufactures another hormone called glucagon. When glucose levels in the blood are low this hormone is released into the bloodstream and it stimulates the liver to release the stored glucose, thus raising the glucose in the blood.

The Impact on the Individual

It has been estimated that there are more than 750 000 people in the UK with diabetes who do not know they have the condition. The main symptoms are some or all of the following:

- increased thirst,
- urinating more frequently: especially at night,
- extreme tiredness,
- weight loss,
- genital itching,
- regular episodes of thrush,
- blurred vision.

Diabetes that is not controlled can cause many serious long-term health problems, such as damaged blood vessels, which in turn contributes to cardiovascular disease (such as hypertension, heart attack and stroke), kidney disease (nephropathy), eye disease (retinopathy) and nerve disease (neuropathy). Uncontrolled diabetes can also result in blindness and amputation.

People with diabetes who drive must inform the Driving and Vehicle Licensing Agency (DVLA) that they have diabetes.

Although there is no cure for diabetes, individuals with the condition should not be restricted from enjoying a full life. The organisation Diabetes UK works very hard at ending discrimination and ignorance for those with diabetes.

The Impact on the NHS

The NHS spends over 10% of its budget treating diabetes and this figure is set to rise. This is due to what has been described as an 'epidemic' in obesity in Western countries, resulting in huge increases in Type 2 diabetes. Government scientists have predicted that over one-third of Britons can now be classed as obese.

Treatment

Individuals with Type 1 diabetes require insulin therapy. This is administered via injection to replace insulin that the body is not producing. As insulin may be short-, medium- or long-acting; some people may need to inject themselves up to three times a day with an insulin pen, just before meals.

Presently, insulin still needs to be given by injection, and not by mouth, as the digestive juices and enzymes would destroy it before it is able to enter the bloodstream and be effective. New innovations are being developed, such as inhaled insulin formats and under-the-skin insulin-releasing rods.

Treatment for Type 2 diabetes is first managed by lifestyle changes. If these are not effective oral drug therapy will be required. As diabetes is a progressive disease, people with Type 2 diabetes may require insulin eventually.

Everyone with diabetes should eat a diet that is low in fat, sugar and salt and should maintain regular physical activity. This is because during exercise the level of glucose in the blood falls, resulting in insulin levels also falling. The aim is to maintain a steady blood glucose level.

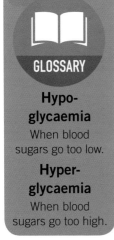

GLOSSARY

Hypo-glycaemia
When blood sugars go too low.

Hyper-glycaemia
When blood sugars go too high.

Monitoring

Monitoring the blood glucose level is a relatively quick and simple procedure, as long as it is conducted correctly. Whichever kit you use, you will need a measuring device, a test strip, a blood lancing device and a sharps box.

- Wash your own hands prior to starting the test. Use warm soapy water. Dry thoroughly. Put on gloves and apron.
- Wash the patient's hand prior to starting the test. Use sterile water. Dry thoroughly.
- Do not use alcohol wipes as this will interfere with the test.
- Prepare your machine. Check that the test strips have been correctly calibrated to the device (this will be displayed on the device screen).

- Place the test strips in machine (this depends on which type of machine you are using).
- Lance the patient's finger, aiming for a ladybird-sized drop of blood. Wipe off this first drop.
- Gently squeeze the finger (not too hard as this may alter the test reading) to obtain another drop of blood.
- Place this drop of blood on the test strip.
- Read the results according to the manufacturer's instructions.
- Document the results and act on any concerns.

Usually, if the result is less than 3.0 mmol/L or greater than 20 mmol/L a medic will request that a venous sample to sent to the laboratory to confirm hypoglycaemia or hyperglycaemia, but this may vary according to Trust.

Sources of contamination include:

1 newsprint (newspapers contain starch),
2 residual sugars from soft drinks or foods,
3 the tester's own hands (if not wearing gloves).

TEST YOUR KNOWLEDGE

1 What do Combur 5 reagent strips test for?
2 How long can a sample of urine be left standing before it must be discarded and cannot be used for urinalysis?
3 Where should the Hema-screen developer be stored?
4 Where are the correct sampling zones for blood lancing?
5 What is hypoglycaemia?

KEY POINTS

- How to conduct an urinalysis test.
- How to undertake a faecal occult blood test.
- Correct procedures for blood lancing for blood glucose monitoring.
- Blood glucose testing.

Chapter 7
· ·
BLOOD TRANSFUSION

Clinical Skills for Nurses, First Edition. Claire Boyd
© 2013 John Wiley & Sons, Ltd. Published 2013 by John Wiley & Sons Ltd.

LEARNING OUTCOMES

By the end of this chapter you will have an understanding of the theory and practice of performing the clinical skill of blood transfusion.

Blood transfusion is one of the clinical skills student nurses can take part in, but only *part* of the process. This is also considered a mandatory training session, which you will probably receive in your induction to an NHS Trust and you will be expected to update your competency assessments every 2 years.

The main blood groups are:
blood group O,
blood group A,
blood group B,
blood group AB.

There is also an antibody known as D Rhesus antigen, or Rh D. If this antigen is present, your blood group is known as *positive*. If this antigen is not present, your blood group is known as *negative*. The blood groups now look like that of Table 7.1.

Table 7.1 Blood groups

Blood group O positive	**Blood group O negative**
Blood group A positive	**Blood group A negative**
Blood group B positive	**Blood group B negative**
Blood group AB positive	**Blood group AB negative**

Did you know, there are also rare blood groups, such as C, E, K, Fy, JK and S?

The O blood group is often referred to as the universal donor, as we can all receive blood from this group (Table 7.2).

Table 7.2 Blood group donors

Blood group	Blood groups that can be a donor
Blood group O	Blood group O only
Blood group A	Blood group A and O
Blood group B	Blood group B and O
Blood group AB	Blood group A, B and O

To donate blood in the UK you need to be at least 17 years old (or 16 years old with parents' permission). The maximum is 65 years, or 75 years if you have been a regular donor. You must also be at least 49.85 kg in weight. Females may donate three times per year, and males four times per year. Each donation is for approximately 470 mL and just one donation can save up to three people's lives. Four per cent of the population donate their blood, but 98% of us state that 'everyone should donate'.

Strict regulation is in place concerning blood matters, from the Department of Health, the National Patient Safety Agency as well as in the form of various European Directives. Part of this concerns training: those who 'manufacture', collect, transport and store the blood, and those who deliver the products (i.e. drivers) need to receive training.

The Serious Hazards of Transfusion (SHOT) organisation oversees the practice of blood transfusion and collects data across the UK on all transfusion reactions, adverse events or 'near-miss' events. From this we can learn from our mistakes. The SHOT report from 2010 is shown in Figure 7.1.

This SHOT report shows that there was a 29% reduction in incorrect blood components being transfused, but a 13.7% increase in acute transfusion reactions, which equates to 13 deaths in the UK. When I give blood to my patients, and invite them to share any concerns, they seem most concerned about 'catching one of those mad-cow diseases'! But figures tell us that the chances

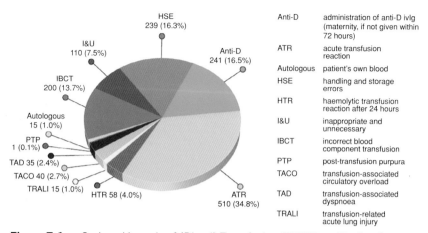

Figure 7.1   Serious Hazards of (Blood) Transfusion (SHOT) audit, showing numbers of cases in 2010. *Source:* Knowles, S. (ed.) and Cohen, H. on behalf of the Serious Hazards of Transfusion (SHOT) Steering Group (2011) *Serious Hazards of Transfusion (SHOT) Report 2010*

of receiving a contaminated blood product are very slight:

1 in 500 000 chance of bacterial contamination,
1 in 670 000 chance of hepatis B infection,
1 in 5 000 000 chance of HIV infection,
1 in 83 000 000 chance of hepatitis C infection.

Only a few cases of vCJD (that's variant Creutzfeldt–Jakob disease, or what the public may call 'mad-cow disease') have been reported after someone has received blood, but doctors must inform patients that this is a risk. Putting this into perspective, we all have a 1 in 200 chance of being involved in a road traffic accident.

Babies' blood products are 'cleaned' and filtered further with a substance called methylene blue, which makes their urine blue and sometimes gives their skin a blue tinge (no wonder their families call them Smurf babies!). The methylene blue inactivates viruses, such as HIV and hepatitis C, and reduces the already small chance of viral transmission even further.

CONSENT AND INFORMATION LEAFLETS

Before a patient received a blood transfusion or a blood product consent must be documented in their notes and a consent form signed. Patients should at this stage have their hospital identification bands in place (usually around their wrists). Figure 7.2 shows what the transfusion record looks like. It is pink in colour. Consent can only be obtained by a doctor or specialist nurse. The patient must also be given a patient information leaflet. As blood is such a precious commodity, the rationale for the patient receiving this 'tissue transplant' must also be written in their notes.

A pre-assessment clinic might wish a patient to increase the iron in their diet prior to being admitted for surgery, to increase their haemoglobin levels.

There are also very strict protocols for the use of blood by surgeons: for example, a surgeon can only order two units of blood for hip-replacement surgery, two units of blood for craniotomy neurosurgery, etc.

It must be remembered that these leaflets come in other languages, as English may not be a patient's first language. The information leaflets are national, but some NHS Trusts may produce their own patient information leaflets.

It should also be remembered that not all patients will be hospital in-patients, and those who are not will require an information sheet to take home after their day-case transfusion.

Other information leaflets concern children and fresh frozen plasma (FFP), which is imported from other countries, usually the USA, and given to anyone born on or after 1 January 1996. This was because of vCJD and the government not knowing who was silently infected with this disease. It is also for this reason that anyone who has received blood or a blood product since 1980 is no longer able to donate their blood. Other information leaflets include guides for parents of children or babies who are receiving blood products.

North Bristol NHS
NHS Trust

BLOOD TRANSFUSION RECORD

It is Trust policy to complete as a minimum:
Section 1: Indication for Transfusion   Section 3: Agreement to Transfusion   Section 4: Prescription
Section 5: Blood Collection   Record of Administration: to record date, time & staff signatures

Hospital..	Affix patient addressograph here or complete below:
Ward/Dept...	**Surname:** ....
Directorate..	**First Name(s):** ....
Consultant..	**Hospital No:** .... **DOB** ....

1. Indication for Transfusion

An Hb threshold of **7g/dl** in otherwise fit patients (8g/dl in older patients and those with known / likely cardiovascular disease) is recommended unless symptomatic or active bleeding.
Transfusion to an Hb above 10g/dl is very rarely indicated unless patient is red cell dependent or a neonate.

Symptoms / signs ....

Diagnosis causing low Hb / anaemia / bleeding...

2. Relevant Medical History

Special considerations..................................

Pre-transfusion Haemoglobin ....g/dl   Blood group ....

Previous transfusion / blood product Yes / No   Previous reaction:Yes / No When: ....

If yes, what and when? ....

3. Agreement to Transfusion

This patient has verbally agreed to a blood transfusion and has received relevant information leaflets or this patient has not provided consent because..

Date .... Staff signature.................................. Print name ....

4. Prescription

Sections 1, 2 and 3 should be completed with prescription, except when 2 & 3 can be done pre-operation
N.B During surgery, prescription on an anaesthetic record is an acceptable alternative

Product & Amount	Date for infusion	Special requirements	Rate	Dr name, sign, date & time

5. Blood Collection (Take blood transfusion record to fridge) *(Requestor & Receiver please sign, and record date & time)*

		Unit 1	Unit 2	Unit 3	Unit 4	Unit 5	Unit 6
Requestor: check patient ID at bedside, patient ID confirmed with collector	Sign:	....	....	....	....	....	....
	Date	....	....	....	....	....	....
	Time	....	....	....	....	....	....
Receiver: take receipt of blood	Sign:	....	....	....	....	....	....
	Date	....	....	....	....	....	....
	Time	....	....	....	....	....	....

Page 1 of 2   Blood Transfusion Record   February 2008   RVJ0694 (LGD)

Figure 7.2 Blood transfusion record. Permission to reproduce this image is granted by North Bristol NHS Trust and University Hospitals Bristol NHS Foundation Trust

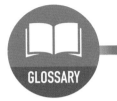

Fresh frozen plasma

The liquid component of human blood that has been frozen for preservation. It is thawed before administration.

variant Creutzfeldt–Jakob disease (vCJD)

A disease thought to be a consequence of eating contaminated beef, related to bovine spongiform encephalopathy (BSE, or so-called mad-cow disease) in UK cattle after 1980. vCJD is very rare, but there is evidence that it may be transmitted from an infected blood donor to a patient via transfusion.

BLOOD TRANSFUSION REQUESTS

Doctors or specialist nurses request blood after consent has been obtained, on a blood transfusion request form. There may be specialist requirements, such as for washed cells, CMV or irradiated blood.

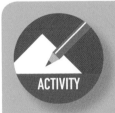

Activity 7.1

Have you ever heard of these blood products? What do you think they mean?

Washed cells
CMV
Irradiated blood

The Blood Transfusion Request Form

The blood transfusion request form must be signed by a doctor or specialist nurse and must contain certain pieces of information: the patient's first name, surname, date of birth and hospital number. Special care must be taken with admissions to hospital with no hospital number, making a patient unable to give identification details.

SAMPLE COLLECTION

A blood sample needs to be collected by venepuncture to perform a cross-match, to check the patient's blood group. Venepuncture (see Chapter 8) can be performed by a doctor, phlebotomist or staff trained in venepuncture, namely:

- registered nurse,
- registered midwife,
- assistant practitioner (or AP),
- healthcare assistant.

Samples for cross-matching are obtained in a blood transfusion tube, known as an EDTA tube, and usually have a red top to identify them as such. Tubes should be labelled at the bedside, and gently inverted to mix the blood with the anticoagulant in the tube. Blood for cross-matching is sent to the same place all samples are sent: the pathology laboratory.

COLLECTING BLOOD THAT HAS BEEN REQUESTED

Pre-Collection Procedure

Before collecting blood, and after confirming that the blood is ready for collection, a cannula must be inserted or checked to establish patency. Check that you have any equipment needed, such as a filtered blood administration set, volumetric pump or blood warmer, if required. Baseline observations must also now be taken. These are:

- temperature,
- pulse,
- blood pressure,
- respiratory rate.

Now go back to the blood transfusion record and you will see that the requestor needs to sign, at the bottom of the document, that they have sent an individual to collect the blood. The requestor must check that the person they are sending has received blood transfusion training and is up to date with their competency. The person collecting the blood must take this record sheet with them to collect the blood.

Collection Procedure

As stated, this requires appropriately trained staff.

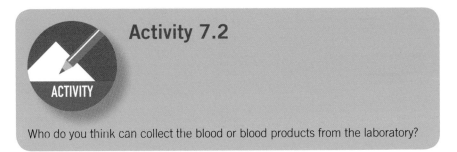

Activity 7.2

ACTIVITY

Who do you think can collect the blood or blood products from the laboratory?

Before you open the fridge containing the units of blood, you will need to check the information you have on the blood transfusion record and the blood register, checking that all the details correspond:

- first name,
- surname,
- date of birth,
- hospital number.

Any discrepancies should be reported immediately. Then take the blood, which should have compatibility form attached (first unit only), much like a luggage label.

NOTE: only take *one bag of blood*, even if the patient has been prescribed more than one unit.

Operating theatres tend to use specialist cool boxes, which can keep the units cold for up to 6 hours. Only theatres can take more than one unit at a time because of these boxes, and they need to have the blood available during surgical procedures.

Check the blood for any signs of leaks or clots.

Check all the details on the compatibility label and the bag of blood and then sign the bag out in the blood register, stating the time that the blood was removed from the fridge. The blood should be transported to the clinical area in a specialised transit bag, or covered so that it is not on full view to other patients and visitors while being transported.

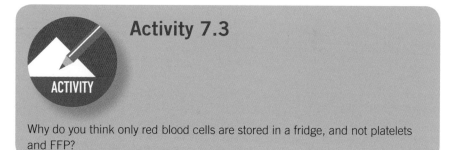

Activity 7.3

ACTIVITY

Why do you think only red blood cells are stored in a fridge, and not platelets and FFP?

Receipt of Blood

Take the blood back to the clinical area and hand to the requestor. The person taking receipt of the unit should check the patient's details on the compatibility label, compatibility report form and the blood transfusion record. They should then sign the blood transfusion record and record the date and time.

COLD-CHAIN REQUIREMENTS

The cold chain relates to the storage and temperature of blood and blood products, and is strictly monitored.

- *Red blood cells* are stored at 2–6°C for 35 days. They must be returned to the fridge within 30 minutes. They require a filtered transfusion administration set.
- *Platelets* are kept at 20–24°C for 5 days in the laboratory and gently agitated. Transfusion must be commenced as soon as possible. They require a special platelet administration set.
- *Fresh frozen plasma* can be kept at −30°C for 2 years. They are thawed in the laboratory by blood bank staff. Infusion should be started immediately once thawed.

PREPARATION/ADMINISTRATION

Some clinical areas require two trained staff to undertake this procedure, while other Trusts may require one trained member of staff to perform this clinical skill. This trained and competent staff member must be a:

- doctor,
- registered nurse,
- registered midwife,
- operating department practitioner.

Student nurses and student operating department practitioners (ODPs) can often check as a third person, but cannot sign any of the paperwork.

The checker(s) should:

- check the patients identification details against the blood unit, transfusion record and compatibility report form,
- check the documentation: prescription, consent, reason for transfusion and baseline observations on the observation chart,
- check the product issue: blood group, Rhesus D, blood bag number, blood unit, compatibility label, compatibility form,
- check the product integrity and special requirements: leaks, clots, discoloration, expiry date, irradiation, CMV-negative, etc.

PRODUCT SPECIFICATIONS

Figure 7.3 shows a bag of blood group O Rh D-negative blood, which is also labelled as CMV-negative.

Blood is now traced from the vein of the donor to vein of the recipient and the barcodes on the bag represent the audit trial. The National Blood Transfusion Service uses a Pulse Tracking System. All donors are given a unique donation number.

If blood is not special blood, then we will see a red block with 'Not Irradiated' on the bag. If a unit is irradiated then we would see a black block on the bag.

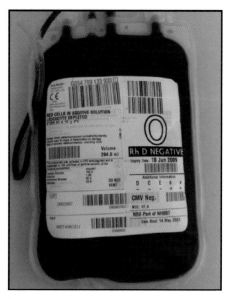

Figure 7.3 Blood bag. Permission to reproduce this image is granted by North Bristol NHS Trust and University Hospitals Bristol NHS Foundation Trust

A blood transfusion record must be completed, including the compatibility form we brought back from the laboratory. This is the form that was attached to the first unit of blood to be transfused.

PRE-TRANSFUSION CHECK

This bedside check is the last one. The patient should give verbal confirmation, checking all the details against the documentation and unit of blood. This compatibility document should be attached to the blood transfusion record sheet.

ADMINISTRATION PROCEDURE

The 'luggage label' is peeled off and attached to a ward register (after signing). Pathology laboratories usually store the originals of this paperwork as legally they must be kept for 30 years. Also, the laboratories will then know where there blood went, as an extra check. Even if the patient received just a few drops from the transfusion, all this paperwork needs to be completed.

Remember to record the start time and unit volume on a fluid chart for your patient and *never* add any drugs to a bag of blood. The rate of transfusion should be monitored, as per the prescription.

The filtered blood administration set/platelet administration set should be changed within 12 hours.

The end of the transfusion should be recorded on the compatibility report form and the observation chart. The empty blood bag should be retained for 24 hours, in case of any adverse reaction.

We may need to work out a drip rate manually, and will therefore need to know the formula for this, in case we can't locate a machine for any reason. We will first need to know how many millilitres of fluid the bag contains and then the length of time that the prescription must take to go through, such as 450 mL and 3 hours. Blood administration sets deliver 15 drops/mL. This is the formula we use:

Rate of transfusion =

$$\frac{\text{volume}}{\text{time in hours}} \times \frac{\text{drops per millilitre}}{60 \text{ minutes}}$$

So, we have:

$$\frac{450 \text{ mL}}{3 \text{ hours}} \times \frac{15 \text{ drops/mL}}{60 \text{ minutes}}$$

$$= 37.5 \text{ drops per minute}$$

This is 450 divided by 3 multiplied by 15 divided by 60. Let a calculator do the work for you. This means that to get the bag of blood through in the prescribed time we need to set the drip rate to 38 drops per minute.

MONITORING PROCEDURE

When the blood or blood product has been started the patient needs to be watched while the first few millilitres are administered. We are looking for any adverse reactions.

The patient needs to be informed that they need to report any shivering, pain, rash, flushing, anxiety, shortness of breath or generally feeling unwell.

Blood transfusion observations are performed *before* the transfusion, *within 15 minutes* of the transfusion going through and at the *end* of the transfusion. This is for every bag or product being transfused. We need to record:

- temperature,
- pulse,
- blood pressure,
- respiratory rate.

Unconscious patients and patients being transfused will need to be monitored more regularly.

Staff who can monitor the patient during the procedure:

- doctor/clinical site manager,
- registered nurse/midwife,
- operating department practitioner/assistant,
- assistant practitioner,
- student nurse/midwife/operating department practitioner or trainee assistant practitioner,
- Band 3 healthcare assistant (HCA).

WHAT TO DO IF THE PATIENT EXPERIENCES AN ADVERSE REACTION

If there is a 1°C rise in the patient's temperature, *stop transfusion immediately!*

- Contact a doctor
- Check the compatibility label with the patient's identification band

- Record a full set of observations
- Reassure the patient
- Record the adverse reaction in the patient notes

If transfusion is discontinued by a medic:

- the reaction must be reported to the blood bank,
- a transfusion reaction form and an Accident and Incident Management System (AIMS) form must be completed

The medic may prescribe antihistamines, paracetamol and to recommence with the transfusion, but at a slower rate.

SAFETY

For safety reasons routine blood transfusions should be administered between the hours of 08:00 and 20:00. This is because there are more staff on duty to observe for any adverse reactions during the daytime, and visible signs such as rashes are easier to spot in daylight.

TEST YOUR KNOWLEDGE

1 What observations need to be carried out for a blood transfusion and when?
2 What is a clinical indicator that the patient is having an adverse reaction to the transfusion?

KEY POINTS

- Understanding blood groups.
- Blood transfusion documents and information leaflets.
- Blood-collection procedures.
- Cold-chain requirements.
- Product specifications.
- Pre- and post-transfusion checks.

Chapter 8
VENEPUNCTURE

Clinical Skills for Nurses, First Edition. Claire Boyd
© 2013 John Wiley & Sons, Ltd. Published 2013 by John Wiley & Sons Ltd.

LEARNING OUTCOMES

By the end of this chapter you will have an understanding of the theory and practice of performing the clinical skill of venepuncture.

WHAT IS VENEPUNCTURE?

The term venepuncture is exactly what the word suggests: entering a vein with a needle, by which we can obtain a sample of blood. It is one of the most commonly performed invasive procedures performed in the healthcare setting. Figure 8.1 shows this procedure being performed.

In the healthcare environment there are many different makes of equipment for venepuncture: the BD Vacutainer system and the Monovette system are just two. Whichever system is used, it must be one designed for the purpose: a needle and syringe *should not* be used generally, although it is accepted practice in many neonatal areas and for some medics.

The collection bottles are colour-coded according to the blood test to be carried out and the additives contained in the tube; for example serum gel, heparin, etc. Gloves should be worn when carrying out the venepuncture

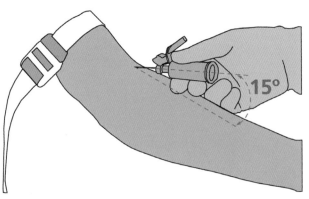

Figure 8.1 The venepuncture procedure. Reproduced with kind permission from BD Diagnostics

procedure, adhering as closely to possible to the aseptic technique. It is also considered best practice for practitioners to check their hepatitis vaccine status to confirm that they are up to date with this immunisation.

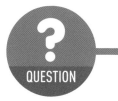

Question 8.1   What do you think are the four main reasons the clinical skill of venepuncture is performed?

COMMON BLOOD TESTS

Venepuncture can be undertaken to obtain a blood sample for testing.

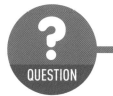

Question 8.2   Name four of the common blood tests.

Full Blood Count

This is one of the most common blood tests and is usually carried out as part of a routine check. Usually the haematology laboratory will divide the full blood count, or FBC, into five results, as follows:

1   *Red blood cell count*: erythrocytes are the most abundant cell type in the blood. By calculating their concentration it is possible to identify whether the patient is anaemic (low concentration) or polycythaemic (high concentration).
2   *Haemoglobin concentration*: the oxygen-carrying component of erythrocytes. If this concentration is low, it is usually an indicator of anaemia.
3   *White cell count*: white blood cells, or leucocytes, form part of the body's defence against infections. They are normally found in low concentrations unless an infection is present, when their number increases.

4 *Differential blood count*: this identifies the concentrations of white blood cells, of which there are five types:
- neutrophils (comprising 50–70% of leucocytes),
- lymphocytes (20–40%),
- monocytes (3–8%),
- eosinophils (2–4 %),
- basophils (0.5–1%).

5 *Platelet count*: an integral part of the clotting system, platelets basically plug the hole when bleeding occurs.

Erythrocyte Sedimentation Rate (ESR)

This is the measurement of the erythrocyte settling rate in anticoagulated blood. Tissue destruction and inflammatory conditions can cause a raised ESR. This result can be very useful in assessing the degree of disease.

C Reactive Proteins (CRP)

This has a similar function as the ESR and is used to monitor the acute phase response of many infections. In response to bacterial infection, trauma, tissue damage and inflammation these levels will rise dramatically.

Liver Function Test (LFT)

This comprises of a number of tests to allow detection of liver disease, placing liver disease into specific category and monitoring the progression of the disease.

Urea and Electrolytes (U&E)

Urea measured in a blood serum sample allows monitoring of kidney and liver function. Urea is the waste product resulting from protein metabolism. Proteins are boken down by digestion into amino acids, which are then sent to the liver. The liver breaks them down further resulting in ammonia, which is toxic to the human body.

High urea levels could indicate:

- renal disease,
- urinary obstruction,

- shock,
- congestive heart failure,
- burns.

Low urea levels could indicate:

- liver failure,
- pregnancy,
- over-hydration,
- starvation.

Electrolytes include:

- sodium,
- potassium,
- chloride,
- bicarbonate,
- creatinine.

Partial Thromboplastin Time (aPTT)

This measures the plasma coagulation factors of the intrinsic pathway, derived from the reagents used in the test to initiate the reaction (partial thromboplastin activator). The aPTT can be increased by:

- deficiencies of plasma proteins specific to the intrinsic pathway,
- heparin,
- degradation products,
- pathological inhibitors,
- severely overdosed warfarin patients.

Prothrombin Time (PT)

This assesses the activity of the extrinsic pathway of blood coagulation. It can be used to detect abnormalities in plasma coagulation. The time taken for the blood to clot when tissue factor and calcium are added is measured. Abnormalities are associated with:

- anticoagulants,
- liver damage,
- vitamin K deficiency,
- overdoses of warfarin.

International Normalised Ratio (INR)

INR, or International Normalized Ratio, is a measurement of blood clotting time. The higher the INR, the longer it will take for your blood to clot. It was introduced by the World Health Organization to provide a common basis for interpretation of prothrombin time. INR is calculated from the patient's PT ratio and a parameter called the International Sensitivity Index (ISI). This accounts for differences in manufacturers' standard samples so that INRs are comparable between laboratories.

Calcium

This is the fifth most common element in the human body. Plasma calcium is necessary for maintaining a normal heart rhythm, the functioning of neurons and muscle contraction, and is involved in the coagulation of blood.

Low plasma calcium levels (hypocalcaemia) may indicate:

- low levels of parathyroid hormone,
- vitamin D deficiency,
- kidney damage,
- certain bone diseases,
- low calcium intake in the diet.

High plasma calcium levels (hypercalcaemia) may indicate:

- overdose of vitamin D,
- increased levels of parathyroid hormone,
- certain cancers,
- high levels of calcium in the diet.

Cholesterol

Cholesterol is a major component of cell membranes; it is excreted in bile or metabolised in bile acids. High levels of cholesterol in the blood can cause severe problems to the arterial and venous systems, building up on vessels and causing inflammation, scarring and eventual blockage of the vessel.

Glucose

Glucose is a simple monosaccharide produced as a result of the digestion of starch/sucrose. The level of glucose in the body is highly regulated by the endocrine function of the pancreas. By monitoring the blood glucose level it is possible to detect whether the patient has poor glucose-level control. A high level (hyperglycaemia) may indicate diabetes.

POLICIES, PROCEDURES AND GUIDELINES

When undertaking the clinical skill of venepuncture, staff must have undertaken specialised training and had assessment for competency. Staff should also be familiar with their local policy for venepuncture, and other relevant policies and acts around:

- sharps handling and disposal,
- informed consent,
- Mental Capacity Act,
- handling and transportation of pathology specimens,
- blood transfusion,
- waste management.

VICARIOUS LIABILITY

It is important to work within your own boundaries, otherwise you may be breaking vicarious liability, which is a legal term defined as:

> ...the principle by which a practitioner's employer will take liability for the actions and omissions of the employee as long as they are acting within their job description and boundaries approved by the employer. (Tilley and Watson 2008)

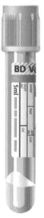

KEEPING UPDATED

After attending a study session on venepuncture, or having completed a recognised e-learning package to your area, certification and assessment documentation should be kept in a portfolio as evidence. As with all clinical skills, this skill should be revisited on a regular basis to keep yourself updated. This may take the form of self-directed learning or by attending a clinical skills update session at your workplace.

EQUIPMENT USED FOR VENEPUNCTURE

The equipment used for obtaining the blood sample depends on the system you are using: this may be a bottle with a coloured top and needle, or, if using the BD Vacutainer system, a blood collection holder, bottle and needle (see Figure 8.2). Some of the newer systems now have the needle and holder integrated, into which the blood bottle is pushed into and punctured. The needle is then covered with a plastic cuff at the end of the procedure as a safety measure to cut down on sharps injuries (see Figure 8.3).

WRITTEN REQUESTS

In the hospital setting a request form will need to be completed by a nurse practitioner or medic, requesting the blood sample needing to be obtained. Requests for blood transfusions will also need to be completed prior to collecting the sample (see Chapter 7). An example of one of these request forms can be seen in Figure 8.4.

Figure 8.2 The BD Vacutainer system. Reproduced with kind permission from BD Diagnostics

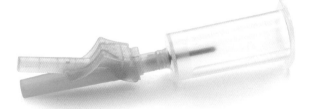

Figure 8.3 A safety-cuffed venepuncture system. Reproduced with kind permission from BD Diagnostics

NORTH BRISTOL NHS TRUST DEPARTMENT OF BLOOD TRANSFUSION						Requesting Doctor .... Bleep No. ....

NORTH BRISTOL NHS TRUST
DEPARTMENT OF BLOOD TRANSFUSION

NHS No. / Hospital No. including Hospital prefix

Surname   Please place approved Addressograph in this area

Forename

D.O.B.   Sex (M/F)   Patient Type

Patients Address inc. Post Code

Consultant / GP Code   Location Code

Clinical Details / Therapy

For Laboratory Use			Inoculation Risk? YES ☐ NO ☐			
				RT	IAG	Time	Initial
ABO	D	Ab Screen				

Frenchay Hospital, Telephone Bristol 0117 340 2780
Southmead Hospital, Telephone Bristol 0117 323 5630

Requesting Doctor .... Bleep No. ....
Signature .... Date & Time ....

Sample Collection
I confirm that I have taken the blood sample for this request in accordance with the NBT Policy, (Summary overleaf) and labelled in the presence of the patient. I have confirmed the patients identity both verbally and with the wristband where available.

Name .... Signature ....
Date and Time .... / .... / .... : ....

☐ Group and Hold

☐ X-Match

Product [   ]   No of Units [   ]

Date & Time required

☐ D D ☐ M M ☐ Y Y ☐ H H ☐ M M

Patient requires Special Blood Products? Y / N

If Yes Give Details ....

☐ Foetal Leak

Other Requests ....

Previously Transfused? (Y/N) ....

When? ....

Any reactions? ....

Blood Group ....

Any irregular antibodies? ....

Most recent Hb ....

Figure 8.4 Blood sample request form for blood transfusion. Permission to reproduce this image is granted by North Bristol NHS Trust and University Hospitals Bristol NHS Foundation Trust

AVAILABLE VEINS

Blood samples are ideally obtained from the median cubital vein across the antecubital fossa (where the arm bends). It is important that health carers performing the clinical skill of venepuncture have an understanding of this basic anatomy in order not to stab an artery with the needle. So, you may wish to look up the blood vessels in the arm.

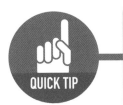

QUICK TIP

Arteries are the same side as the little finger. Go up the arm from the little finger, feel for a pulse in the antecubital fossa and then go to the opposite side along this crease until you feel the blood vessel with no pulse. Voilà: a vein!

The antecubital fossa is the approved site for venepuncture because it is able to tolerate repeat samples, is the most stable vein, is one of the larger veins, is close to the surface of the body and is said to be the least sensitive area.

Medics and other specialist health carers sometimes obtain blood samples from the groin, feet or neck, but this is certainly not routine. Obtaining a sample from the feet may cause the patient to experience an air embolism or other complication, such as necrosis in patients with diabetes.

Vein Anatomy

Veins have three layers. They also contain valves, which help, with muscle movement, to shunt the blood back towards the heart. Connective tissue helps to keep the veins in place. As we get older, there may be a loss of connective tissue, and the vessels can become quite mobile and will require some traction (downwards pulling) to be stabilised and straightened. As valves are sited all along the veins we may inadvertently hit one, which will cause the patient some pain. If this happens then remove the needle and dispose of it, apologise to the patient and explain what has happened and that the vein will repair itself.

The Ideal Vein

Veins do not have a pulse and will refill when depressed. The vein needs to be soft and bouncy, and ideally it should be well supported by subcutaneous tissue. Sometimes the vein may be visible. It is always considered good practice to ask the patient's preference about which arm to use, and they may also know which arm is better for giving blood.

The Poor Vein

When selecting the vein for venepuncture we should try to avoid mobile, hard and inflamed or painful veins. Also stay away from bruised or infected areas. We should avoid areas where intravenous fluids or medication are being transfused, opting for the opposite arm.

Extra skill will be required by the health carer for patients with damaged veins, such as intravenous drug abusers.

Vein Selection

Prior to selecting the vein for venepuncture we will need to know the clinical status of our patient. For example, if a patient (male or female) has undergone breast surgery they may be experiencing lymphoedema (lymph drainage problems) so we will need to obtain our sample from the other, non-affected arm. If this patient has undergone a double mastectomy, and for patients who have peripherally shut down, it is more usual for medics or specialised staff to perform the venepuncture.

In addition, patients on medication that slows down the clotting cascade will require more pressure on the puncture site as the bleeding will take longer to stop when the needle is removed from the vein. It is not correct to say that drugs such as heparin, aspirin and warfarin 'thin the blood': it is the clotting factor that is affected.

It is important to involve the patient in the venepuncture procedure and to try to put them at their ease and gain their co-operation. Listen to the patient: have they had this procedure performed previously? Ask 'How was it for you?' This way we are gathering information on the patient and the way in which we have perfomed the technique (to be forewarned is to be forearmed!).

It is very difficult to obtain a blood sample from a patient who is dehydrated and from those with difficult-to-locate veins (such as obese patients), so it is important to know your limitations and not attempt the procedure if you do not have the competence. It is usual to only make two attempts at venepuncturing, or three in an emergency.

SKIN CLEANING

The venepuncture site should be cleaned thoroughly with a cleaning agent, such as with a 70% isopropyl alcohol/2% chlorhexidine wipe (e.g. a Clinell swab) or a 70% isopropyl alcohol wipe (e.g. Steret). It must then be left to dry. Povidine iodine 10% must be used as an alternative if the patient is sensitive to chlorhexidine. It is recommended that the site is not re-palpated after cleansing, although this maybe necessary if the patient's vein is very difficult to find.

ORDER OF DRAW

The order of draw is in what order the blood samples should be collected. Each of the colour-topped bottles contain chemicals to prevent clotting of the sample, and some of these chemicals may dribble out and contaminate the next sample.

Figure 8.5 shows an example of the order of draw, but it is important to establish the order of draw for the area in which you are collecting samples and for the system of venepuncture that you are using.

LABELLING THE TUBES

Many sampling errors are made by the venepuncture sample not being labelled at the bedside. Therefore it is good practice to label the tubes as soon as the sample has been taken, and not to get distracted. Patients should have their identity bands checked against the documentation to establish that the correct patient is being venepunctured. The patient should also be asked to verbally state their name and date of birth, if possible.

Community situations have their own safety measures in place. For instance, care homes often have residents' pictures on the bedroom doors and in health centres patients attend scheduled appointments.

Any biohazard specimens should be well labelled and are usually double-bagged.

POTASSIUM AND CALCIUM

When obtaining potassium or calcium samples a tourniquet should not be used. This is because a tourniquet slows the movement of blood and alters the chemicals obtained in the sample, showing higher readings. If a tourniquet is used, then it is usual to insert the needle into the vein, remove the tourniquet and wait for approximately 1 minute before obtaining the blood sample. The pathology laboratory should then be informed that a tourniquet was used.

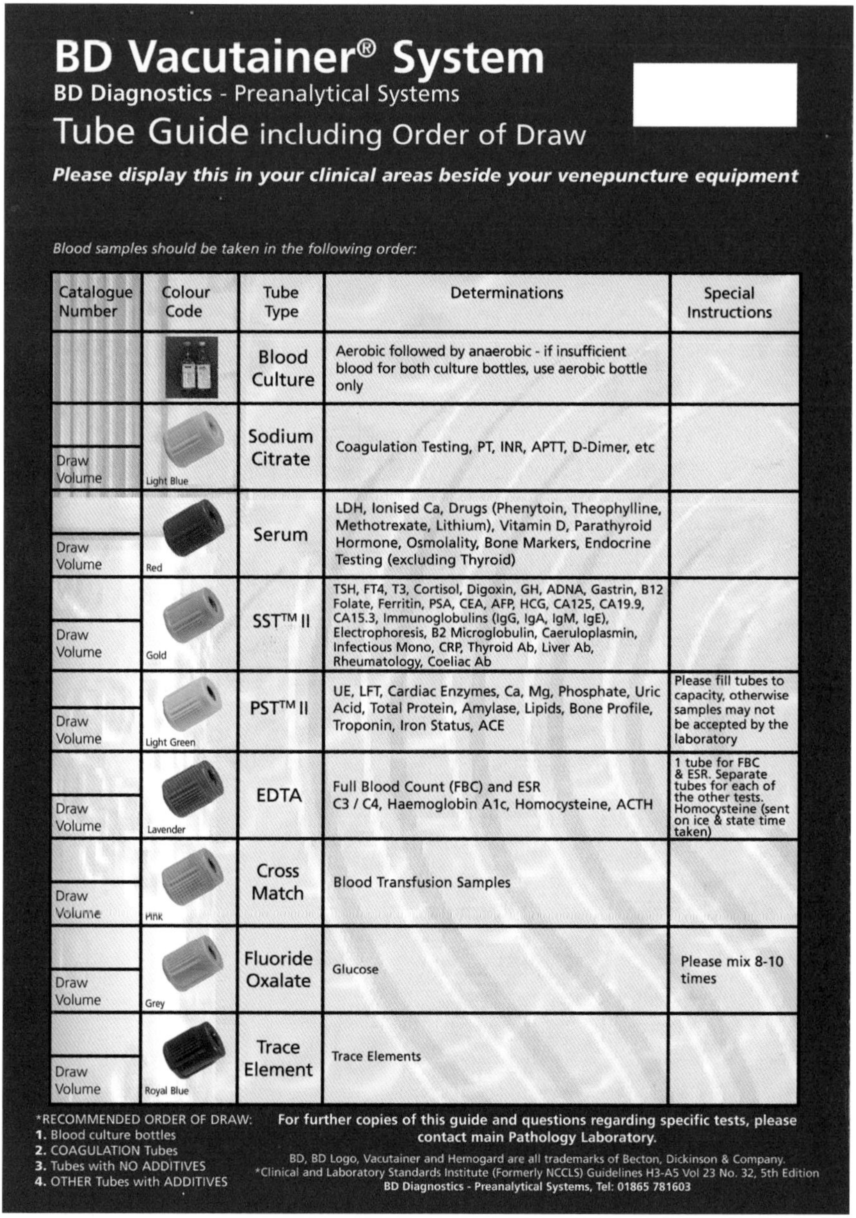

BD Vacutainer® System

BD Diagnostics - Preanalytical Systems

Tube Guide including Order of Draw

Please display this in your clinical areas beside your venepuncture equipment

Blood samples should be taken in the following order:

Catalogue Number	Colour Code	Tube Type	Determinations	Special Instructions
		Blood Culture	Aerobic followed by anaerobic - if insufficient blood for both culture bottles, use aerobic bottle only	
Draw Volume	Light Blue	Sodium Citrate	Coagulation Testing, PT, INR, APTT, D-Dimer, etc	
Draw Volume	Red	Serum	LDH, Ionised Ca, Drugs (Phenytoin, Theophylline, Methotrexate, Lithium), Vitamin D, Parathyroid Hormone, Osmolality, Bone Markers, Endocrine Testing (excluding Thyroid)	
Draw Volume	Gold	SST™ II	TSH, FT4, T3, Cortisol, Digoxin, GH, ADNA, Gastrin, B12 Folate, Ferritin, PSA, CEA, AFP, HCG, CA125, CA19.9, CA15.3, Immunoglobulins (IgG, IgA, IgM, IgE), Electrophoresis, B2 Microglobulin, Caeruloplasmin, Infectious Mono, CRP, Thyroid Ab, Liver Ab, Rheumatology, Coeliac Ab	
Draw Volume	Light Green	PST™ II	UE, LFT, Cardiac Enzymes, Ca, Mg, Phosphate, Uric Acid, Total Protein, Amylase, Lipids, Bone Profile, Troponin, Iron Status, ACE	Please fill tubes to capacity, otherwise samples may not be accepted by the laboratory
Draw Volume	Lavender	EDTA	Full Blood Count (FBC) and ESR C3 / C4, Haemoglobin A1c, Homocysteine, ACTH	1 tube for FBC & ESR. Separate tubes for each of the other tests. Homocysteine (sent on ice & state time taken)
Draw Volume	Pink	Cross Match	Blood Transfusion Samples	
Draw Volume	Grey	Fluoride Oxalate	Glucose	Please mix 8-10 times
Draw Volume	Royal Blue	Trace Element	Trace Elements	

*RECOMMENDED ORDER OF DRAW:
1. Blood culture bottles
2. COAGULATION Tubes
3. Tubes with NO ADDITIVES
4. OTHER Tubes with ADDITIVES

For further copies of this guide and questions regarding specific tests, please contact main Pathology Laboratory.

BD, BD Logo, Vacutainer and Hemogard are all trademarks of Becton, Dickinson & Company.
*Clinical and Laboratory Standards Institute (Formerly NCCLS) Guidelines H3-A5 Vol 23 No. 32, 5th Edition
BD Diagnostics - Preanalytical Systems, Tel: 01865 781603

Figure 8.5 BD order of draw chart. Reproduced with kind permission from BD Diagnostics

PAEDIATRICS

Special precautions apply in children's nursing and special care baby units (neonatal intensive care, or NICU): in the NICU areas of many NHS Trusts no student doctors, healthcare assistants or radiographers may undertake venepuncture. In addition, tourniquets are also not used in NICU.

For infants weighing less than 1.5 kg or aged less than 30 weeks, 0.05% chlorhexidine must be used. For infants weighing more than 1.5 kg or aged more than 30 weeks 0.5% chlorhexidine must be used.

PROBLEMS ASSOCIATED WITH VENEPUNCTURE

The main problems associated with venepuncture, apart from not being able to locate the vein in the first place, are:

- haematoma/bruising,
- excessive pain,
- needlestick injury,
- fainting,
- nerve damage,
- infection,
- hardening of the veins,
- haemorrhage,
- blood spillage,
- arterial stab, i.e. stabbing an artery instead of the intended vein,
- embolism: air getting into bodily system.

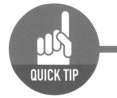

QUICK TIP

Don't panic if you do stab an artery. *Call for help*, put pressure on the site and reassure your patient.

Needlestick Injury

If you inadvertently stab yourself with a used needle you will need to:

1 encourage the wound to bleed by squeezing,
2 wash it thoroughly with running water,
3 cover the wound with a waterproof dressing,
4 call your local needlestick injury hotline and/or occupational health to report the injury,
5 inform your manager/mentor and complete an accident form.

USING A TOURNIQUET

Placing a tourniquet approximately 10 cm above the intended puncture site creates stasis of the blood (i.e. slows down the blood flow). Tourniquets come in different designs and it is important to adhere to infection-control principles and ideally use single-use tourniquets only to minimise spread of infection. Figure 8.6 shows a tourniquet in place.

Two fingers are placed under the tourniquet when tying or buckling up, to create the right amount of stasis, and so as

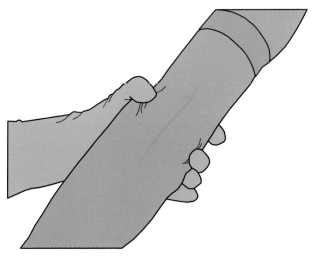

Figure 8.6 A tourniquet in place to create stasis of blood flow. Reproduced with kind permission from BD Diagnostics

not to cause pinching of the skin. Always check whether the tourniquet contains latex to protect your latex-sensitive patients.

The tourniquet should be moved as soon as possible, for if kept on too long it may cause nerve damage. Blood pressure cuffs can also be used, up to the pressure of approximately 80 mmHg.

Catheter tubes and gloves must never be used as a tourniquet, as this is not what they were designed for! Squeezing the area with two hands is also not best practice.

GUIDELINES FOR THE VENEPUNCTURE PROCEDURE

Equipment needed

Gloves (and plastic apron if contamination is unavoidable or patient is an infection risk)

Cleaning agent: a 70% isopropyl alcohol/2% chlorhexidine wipe (e.g. a Clinell swab; 2% chlorhexidine is for adults: use 0.05% for infants weighing less than 1.5 kg and 0.5% for those more than 1.5 kg), a 70% isopropyl alcohol wipe (e.g. Steret) or povidine iodine 10% (if the patient is sensitive to chlorhexidine)

Needle

Tubes

Cotton wool balls

Tourniquet (preferably disposable)

Plastic sharps tray

Plaster (if appropriate)

Sharps box

Procedure	
1	Explain the procedure to the patient, gaining valid consent.
2	Check that the identity of the patient matches the details on the request form or electronic register.
3	Gather equipment together on a plastic tray with the sharps bin, and take to the bedside.
4	Assist that patient into an appropriate position to allow access to the limb for venepuncture.
5	Arrange the limb so that the patient is comfortable.
6	Apply the tourniquet, assess and select the appropriate vein and release the tourniquet.

7	Put on the plastic apron. Wash your hands using soap and water and the six-step hand-decontamination technique.
8	Open the outer plastic packaging and prepare equipment.
9	Put on the gloves.
10	Clean the patient's skin and the selected vein thoroughly. Allow to dry for 30 seconds. Do not re-palpate the vein or touch the skin afterwards.
11	Re-apply the tourniquet.
12	Remove the needle's sheath and inspect the needle for any faults.
13	Anchor the vein by applying manual traction on the skin a few centimeters below the proposed site of insertion.
14	Ensure the needle is in the bevel-up position and insert the needle through the skin at the selected angle according to the depth of the vein.
15	Reduce the angle of descent of the needle as soon as the vein has been punctured.
16	Pull back the plunger or leave until the required amount of blood is obtained by vacuum, depending on system being used.
17	Remove the first tube while keeping the needle still; apply any further tubes in accordance with the order of draw.
18	When all required samples are obtained, release the tourniquet.
19	Remove the needle, but do not apply pressure until the needle has been fully removed.
20	Apply digital pressure directly over the puncture site.
21	Dispose of the needle into sharps container.
22	Gently the invert tubes.
23	Label the tubes with all relevant details.
24	Observe the site for signs of swelling or leakage, and ask the patient if any discomfort or pain is felt.
25	Apply dressing, if appropriate.
26	Discard waste in appropriate waste bins.
27	Remove gloves and apron, and wash hands.
28	Document date, time, site and reason for venepuncture in patient's record and send off the sample(s).

TEST YOUR KNOWLEDGE

1 What is the maximum time that practitioners undertaking venepuncture are advised that tourniquets can stay *in situ*?
2 Why should patients not clench their fists too hard (to bring up the veins) during venepuncture?
3 In relation to venepuncture, what is order of draw?
4 At what age are individuals presumed to be able to give consent?
5 Practitioners undertaking venepuncture are advised by occupational health to have been immunised against what?
6 Before venepuncture is attempted, what must be obtained from the patient?
7 Blood samples for pre-blood transfusion compatibility testing can be taken by which healthcare personnel?
8 If a blood sample is ascertained to monitor drug levels, what must be recorded?

KEY POINTS

- Rationale for the venepuncture procedure.
- Common blood tests.
- Vein selection for venepuncture.
- Order of draw.
- Problems associated with venepuncture.
- The venepuncture procedure.

Chapter 9

· ·

PERIPHERAL CANNULATION

Clinical Skills for Nurses, First Edition. Claire Boyd

© 2013 John Wiley & Sons, Ltd. Published 2013 by John Wiley & Sons Ltd.

LEARNING OUTCOMES

By the end of this chapter you will have an understanding of the theory and practice of performing the clinical skill of cannulation.

Peripheral venous cannulation is when a plastic or metal tube is inserted into a peripheral vein for intravenous (IV) therapy, such as IV fluids and/or drugs or the transfusion of blood products. A further indication of use is also for the administration of dyes and contrast media during clinical investigations. Some acute areas also insert a device for prophylactic reasons, 'just in case'.

The device used is a peripheral venous catheter (PVC), commonly referred to as a cannula. These devices come in different colour-coded sizes – known as the gauge size – and many different styles, depending on manufacturer. Figure 9.1 shows a typical PVC device: blood samples can be obtained from this type of PVC, but usually only immediately after it has been inserted. However, if a patient has very poor veins and a blood sample cannot be obtained from any other site it is usually permitted, but you will need to check that this is accepted practice in your area. In this case, the first 5 mL of blood will

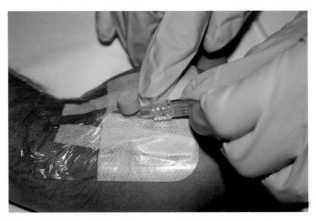

Figure 9.1 A peripheral venous catheter (PVC) device

need to be discarded and the PVC flushed after the procedure.

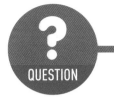

Question 9.1   For what reasons would you need to insert a PVC device? List five.

SELECTION OF AN APPROPRIATE CANNULA

A PVC must never totally occlude a vein: the smallest cannula should be selected. However, if our patient is critically ill and the situation is an emergency, for example during hypovolaemic shock, this rule does not apply. Then we insert a larger device to 'push the fluids' into the patient's system as quickly as possible for rapid treatment.

We also need to think about the intended infusate and at what speed this fluid needs to 'go through'. This will have a bearing on our cannula choice.

A PVC device should usually be replaced after 72 hours (3 days), but should be flushed, usually with 0.9% sodium chloride every 4–6 hours (see Flushing, page 156).

Table 9.1 Cannula selection

Colour	Common applications	Size gauge	Approximate flow rate (L/hour)		
			Crystalloid	Plasma	Blood
Orange	Used in theatres or emergency for rapid transfusion of blood or viscous fluids	14 G	16.2	13.5	10.3
Grey	Used in theatres or emergency for rapid transfusion of blood or viscous fluids	16 G	10.8	9.4	7.1
White	Blood transfusions, rapid infusion of large volumes of viscous liquids	17 G	7.5	6.5	4.6

(continued)

Table 9.1 *(Continued)*

Colour	Common applications	Size gauge	Approximate flow rate (L/hour)		
			Crystalloid	Plasma	Blood
Green	Blood transfusions, parenteral nutrition, stem cell harvesting and cell separation, large volumes of fluids	18 G	4.8	4.1	2.7
Pink	Blood transfusions, large volumes of fluids	20 G	3.2	2.9	1.9
Blue	Blood transfusions, most medications and fluids	22 G	1.9	1.7	1.1
Yellow	Medications, short term infusions, fragile veins, children	24 G	0.8	0.7	0.5
Purple	Neonatal	26 G	0.8	0.7	0.5

Reproduced with kind permission of BD Diagnostics.

Traditionally a green cannula (18 gauge) was used to infuse blood as it was thought that a smaller gauge would damage the red blood cells. Most bags of blood are between 300 and 400 mL and need to be administered within 3–4 hours. We can see from Table 9.1 that in an hour we can infuse up to 2700 mL (or 2.7 litres) of blood via a green cannula (18 gauge, or 18 G). Even in paediatrics we can run through 500 mL of blood via a yellow (24 gauge) and purple (26 gauge) cannula with this make of cannula. Note: other manufacturers' colour of gauge sizes may vary.

THE PVC DEVICE

The cannula comes in three parts. Before use we need to check the packaging, which will tell us whether the device is latex-free and the fact that it is single use. This packaging will also show us the gauge size, lot number and expiry date as well as how many millilitres per minute can be infused through the device.

APPROVED SITE

It is usual to site a cannula on the back of the hand and then work your way up to the antecubital fossa (see Chapter 8). Doctors and some specialist nurses may cannulate in the legs and feet, but this is more problematic as there is more chance of causing an air embolism at these sites, so nurses are generally not permitted to use them. In addition, patients with diabetes may experience more complications in the leg and feet, due to the small-fibre neuropathic damage that this disease causes.

Points of flexion should be avoided and the cannula secured with an appropriate dressing to avoid movement of the device.

VEIN SELECTION

Vein selection is by the same procedures as described for venepuncture (see Chapter 8), not forgetting to ask whether our patient has had this procedure before; in other words, involving them in the process.

Mobile veins on the back of the hands can be difficult to cannulate. In this case we need to add a little traction, meaning that the vein should be pulled taut. It is for this reason that it is always best to practice your technique on patients who are a little easier to cannulate, until you become more experienced.

NUMBER OF ATTEMPTS

It is usual to allow only two attempts when trying to insert a cannula. It is then best to ask someone else to cannulate the patient. Of course, in an emergency or if someone has very difficult veins more than two attempts are often permitted.

SKIN PREPARATION

The site of cannulation should be cleaned thoroughly using a cleaning agent, such as 70% isopropyl alcohol/2% chlorhexidine wipe (e.g. a Clinell swab) or a 70% isopropyl alcohol wipe (e.g. Steret). The skin should be cleaned for about 30 seconds and then left to dry for a further 30 seconds.

ASEPSIS

Apron and gloves should be worn during the procedure. If a patient is having IV fluids administered and the set-up needs to be disconnected when going to X-ray, etc., a bung should be used to cover the administration port on the device and the line disconnected. A new line should be set up on the patient's return.

FLUSHING

A PVC device should be flushed, usually with 0.9% sodium chloride, every 4–6 hours. The procedure for this technique is called the **push/pause technique**. Draw up the flush and administer it by injecting approximately 1 mL, then stopping, then pushing in another 1 mL and stopping again. Continue with this process until the flush has been administered in full. The rationale for this procedure is to create many different episodes of turbulence to stop any build-up of clotted blood at the end of the cannula.

Nothing smaller than a 10 mL syringe should be used to flush a cannula, ideally with 10 mL of fluid. With smaller syringes too much pressure may be applied to the vein. Prior to a flush the hub of the cannula should be cleaned, usually with the same substance we use to clean the skin, such as an alcohol wipe: this is known as 'scrubbing the hub'.

DOCUMENTATION

Records must be kept of who inserted the device, where on the body it was and the date on which it was performed. The cannulation site should be inspected every shift and information recorded on the care plan.

All cannula sites should be covered by a transparent dressing so that the site can be inspected for any sign of phlebitis. This visual inspection is called a VIP (for visual inspection of phlebitis) and a score is given to the site area. Figure 9.2 shows a typical cannulation care plan. We can see that for a score of two and above we should resite the cannula.

North Bristol
NHS Trust

Peripheral Cannulae Care Plan

Name		Date of Birth	
Hospital Number		Department	
	Cannula 1	Cannula 2	Cannula 3
Location of Cannula			
Date of Insertion			
Time of Insertion			
Location of Insertion			
Insert by (Print Name)			
Reason for Cannulation			
Size/Colour of Cannula			
Date of Removal			
Time of Removal			
Removed by (Print Name)			

Visual Infusion Phlebitis (VIP) Score
(adopted from Andrew Jackson's VIP score)

Signs		Actions
Intravenous (IV) site appears healthy	0	No sign of phlebitis Observe cannula
Slight pain near IV site or Slight redness near IV site	1	Possible first sign of phlebitis Observe cannula

Two of the following:
   Pain near IV site
   Erythema
   Swelling
	2	Early stage of phlebitis
		Resite cannula

Pain along path of cannula Erythema and Induration	3	Medium stage of phlebitis Resite cannula Consider treatment

All of the following is evident and extensive:
   Pain along path of cannula
   Erythema
   Induration
   Palpable venous cord
	4	Advanced stage of phlebitis or start of thrombophlebitis
		Resite cannula
		Consider treatment

All of the following is evident and extensive:
   Pain along path of cannula
   Erythema
   Induration
   Palpable venous cord
   Pyrexia
	5	Advanced stage of thrombophlebitis
		Initiate treatment
		Resite cannula

Figure 9.2 Peripheral cannulae care plan. Reproduced with permission from North Bristol NHS Trust and University Hospitals Bristol NHS Foundation Trust

PROBLEMS ASSOCIATED WITH CANNULATION

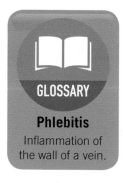

GLOSSARY

Phlebitis

Inflammation of the wall of a vein.

The same problems apply to cannulation as venepuncture, namely infection, pain and nerve damage. Phlebitis is also a potential problem when performing this procedure, and can be caused by:

* *infection*: causing inflammation of the vein,
* *mechanical phlebitis*: caused by the cannula rubbing and irritating the lining of the vein (tunica intima),
* *chemical phlebitis*: caused by the drug being infused, such as strongly alkaline, acidic or hypertonic drugs.

Additional problems are what used to be called 'tissuing', but which should be called **extravasation** or **infiltration** (see Chapter 11).

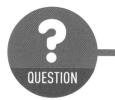

QUESTION

Question 9.2 What do the terms extravasation and infiltration mean?

If a large amount of fluids have infiltrated the surrounding tissues then swelling, pain and nerve damage may occur. Surgery may be required to drain the fluid.

REMOVING THE CANNULA

Cannulae are radio-opaque, meaning that they will show up under X-ray. This is important as we always need to check that we have retrieved the whole device on removal and that none of it has been left behind in the patient's body to migrate and cause damage.

TEST YOUR KNOWLEDGE

1   Can a blood sample be obtained from a cannula?
2   What technique should be used to administer a flush?
3   What is the golden rule of cannul selection?

4   What is the approximate flow rate in litres/hour of a crystalloid fluid in a 22 gauge cannula?

5   What size syringe should we use to flush a cannula?

6   What does VIP stand for?

KEY POINTS

- Selection of an appropriate device.
- Cannula selection.
- Approved sites and vein selection.
- Skin preparation and asepsis.
- Documentation and the VIP score.
- Problems associated with cannulation.

Chapter 10
· · · · · · · · · · · · · · · · · ·
EARLY PATIENT ASSESSMENT AND RESPONSE

Clinical Skills for Nurses, First Edition. Claire Boyd
© 2013 John Wiley & Sons, Ltd. Published 2013 by John Wiley & Sons Ltd.

LEARNING OUTCOMES

By the end of this chapter you will have an understanding of the theory and practice of performing the clinical skill of recognising the deteriorating patient.

In 2007 the National Patient Safety Agency published a report after analysing 576 patient deaths stating that 11% of deaths related to patient deterioration were not recognised or acted upon (National Patient Safety Agency 2007a).

The National Patient Safety Agency report identified four key findings:

* not taking observations,
* not recognising early signs of deterioration,
* not communicating observations causing concern,
* not responding to these concerns appropriately.

From this report strategies for patient safety where put in place, including:

* *SBAR* training programmes, using critical language in clinical areas (SBAR stands for Situation, Background, Assessment, Recommendation),
* *EWS*, or Early Warning Score, using the Bristol Observation Chart,
* *EPAR* training programmes (or Early Patient Assessment and Response), using the ABCDE approach.

SITUATION, BACKGROUND, ASSESSMENT, RECOMMENDATION (SBAR)

This is a communication tool referred to as 'critical language'. The tool is used in the airline business whereby key phrases are understood by all to mean 'stop and listen to me – we have a potential problem'. Put simply, this is

'Doctor, I'm *concerned* about Patient A and would like you to review her *immediately*.'

Of course, medics require more information than this and this is where we get the 'situation, background, assessment and recommendations' bit from:

- *situation*: punchline to be given in 5–10 seconds. No waffling.
- *background*: how did we get here? Admitting diagnosis. Medical history.
- *assessment*: what is the problem? Give ABCDE recording results.
- *recommendation*: what do we need to do?

Here is an example of how the tool is used in practice:

Doctor, I'm concerned about Patient A, who was admitted this morning with a chest infection. I have just assessed her and her vital signs are: BP 192/74, pulse 110 irregular, respirations 30 breaths per minute, temperature 38.4°C, oxygen saturation (SpO$_2$) 93% on 2 L of oxygen therapy, AVPU is V. Her Early Warning Score is 5. Would you like me to increase her oxygen therapy and arrange for an ECG? I would like you to review her immediately. How often would you like vital sign recordings?

Using the SBAR communication tool really does stop you from panicking and keeps you focused. During this communication all the bases were covered: the situation, background, assessment and recommendations.

EARLY WARNING SCORE (EWS)

We looked at the Bristol Observation Chart in Chapter 1 (see Appendix 1). Let's reacquaint ourselves with this document, looking at the two pages of the chart. Each vital sign on the chart generates a score, from 0 to 3. A score of 2 and above generates a *trigger* for action to be implemented, and the second page of the chart shows what action needs to be taken. A score of 4 and above tells us our patient is rather sick and requires an urgent review by the medics.

When speaking to a medic we would use the SBAR communication tool, using concise and relevant language to convey our concerns. Now you can see how the EWS and SBAR are important tools in improving our response to vital signs when a patient first starts to deteriorate.

On the chart, bottom right, is a box saying 'revised trigger'. This is where a consultant or registrar can adjust the trigger score, initiating a response by the care team. This means that where there is usually a call for action on a score of 2 and above, we may now only be required to do this on a score of 4.

Activity 10.1

ACTIVITY

Here's some practice at using the Bristol Observation Chart. You are looking after Sandra Singh. She is 65 years old and had a section of her bowel removed 3 days ago due to a cancerous tumour. She has been stable post-operatively and has not encountered any major problems. She now has a temporary colostomy, which is functioning. She has non-insulin dependent diabetes. Her EWS score has been 0 and her blood glucose levels have been stable.

Sandra is now due her 4-hourly observations. Plot these on a copy of the chart. Her blood glucose is 6.2 mmol/L. What is her EWS score? What are your actions, if any?

Respiratory rate: 23 breaths per minute
Oxygen saturation, SpO_2: 92% (on air)
Blood pressure: 88/50 mmHg
Heart rate: 115 beats per minute (tachycardia)
Neurological response: verbal
Temperature: 37.8°C

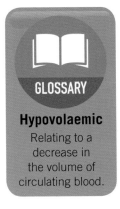

Activity 10.2

Now try communicating all the information you gathered in Activity 10.1 to the medics using the SBAR communications tool.

EARLY PATIENT ASSESSMENT AND RESPONSE (EPAR)

GLOSSARY

Hypovolaemic
Relating to a decrease in the volume of circulating blood.

Did you wonder why Sandra Singh, in Activity 10.1, had started to deteriorate so quickly? She had been sitting up and chatting just 1 hour previously (and boy, can she chat!) and now was only responsive to verbal neurological observations. Well, this was because no one had looked at her wound site (the colostomy) and noticed that she was bleeding profusely from it, and that she was actually hypovolaemic, hence the drop in blood pressure and increase in heart rate.

If you have done first aid you may have used the ABC approach, but in health care we have the ABCDE assessment:

A   Airway
B   Breathing
C   Circulation (including cannulation)
D   Disability and diuresis (drugs and diabetes)
E   Expose and early call for help using SBAR

Airway

The first assessment we perform on our patient is the airway. If the airway is occluded, our patient will die, so we will need to address this immediately and clear the obstruction. We need to check that our patient can talk either normally, in sentences, in words, or whether they are unable to talk or are unresponsive. The assessment includes:

- *looking*: any obvious obstruction such as vomit or foreign objects?
- *feeling*: is the chest rising and falling?
- *listening*: can the patient speak? Any gurgling, wheezing or stridor?
- *smelling*: any smell of alcohol, solvents or ketones?

If the patient is expectorating sputum, this is part of the airway assessment. We need to report on the colour, odour, consistency and amount.

When we are satisfied that the airway is clear we can move on to the breathing assessment.

Breathing

This assessment consists of measuring the respiratory rate. Signs of respiratory deterioration include:

- increased respiratory rate (especially if above 30 breaths per minute),
- oxygen decrease by 3%,
- increasing oxygen requirements,
- increasing EWS score,
- carbon dioxide retention with blood pH below 7.35,
- drowsiness,
- headache,
- tremor.

The breathing assessment requires us to look at the patient for signs of cyanosis around the lips, oral mucosa and nails. We need to observe the depth of breathing and to look for any 'see-saw' chest movements (which may be a sign of a pneumothorax) and for oedema around the face, which may be interfering with the airway.

Our patient may be experiencing dyspnoea with shortness of breath and will assume a position that best facilitates lung expansion: sat forward in their chair, arching back, breathing through the mouth, shoulders forward and nostrils flaring.

If the breathing assessment has not triggered any action based on the EWS score, or any concerns, we can move on to circulation.

Circulation

This assessment includes monitoring the pulse (heart rate) and blood pressure. If our patient is experiencing chest pain, and after we have contacted the medics, we may need to conduct an ECG. The ECG can tell us (in ST elevation) whether muscle damage has occurred, or if ischemia has occurred (in ST depression).

The doctor may wish the patient to have intravenous (IV) access, so a cannula may need to be inserted for crystalloid/colloid fluids to be administered, and other IV drugs.

A **capillary refill** test may be conducted. This is measures the rate at which blood refills empty capillaries.

1   Press firmly on a finger nail to blanch it and count the time it takes for blood to return after the pressure is released.
2   In a normal person, with good cardiac output and digital profusion, capillary refill should take less than 3 seconds.
3   A time of more than 3 seconds is considered a sign of sluggish digital circulation.
4   A time of 5 seconds is considered abnormal.

If the circulation assessment has not triggered any action based on the EWS score, or any concerns, we can move on to disability.

Disability

This assessment has four parts and concerns making neurological observations (the disability component) as well as diuresis, drugs and diabetes.

On our Bristol Observation Chart, if our patient has recorded anything other than alert in the neurological response section we need to conduct a full Glasgow Coma Scale (GCS) assessment.

There are many causes of altered consciousness (Table 10.1).

Table 10.1 Causes of altered consciousness

Profound hypoxaemia	Cerebral hypoperfusion
Hypercapnia	Stroke
Convulsions	Sedatives
Head injury	Hypoglycaemia
Alcohol intoxication	Analgesic drugs
Subarachnoid haemorrhage	Drug overdose

Figure 10.1 shows an example of a neurological observation chart, incorporating the GCS and EWS systems. In short, the GCS looks at the responses of:

- eye opening,
- motor response,
- verbal response.

This document also has *limb movement* and *pupillary assessment* sections. At the bottom of the chart, there are instructions on what to do if the neurological examination is abnormal, the EWS score to add and the actions to take.

Motor Response

This assessment is designed to determine the patient's ability to obey commands and to localise, and to withdraw (or assume abnormal body positions) in response to painful stimuli, such as the trapezium squeeze.

- *Score 6* if the patient can obey a command.
- *Score 5* if the patient localises to central pain. This means that the patient does not respond to verbal stimuli but purposely moves an arm to remove the cause of a central painful stimulus.

Neurological Observation Chart GCS

To be used in conjunction with Bristol Observation Chart

Not to be used on Neuroscience wards

Name: ....

Date of Birth: ....

Hospital No.: ....

Ward: ....

Ensure sections shaded grey are completed after discussion with medical staff requesting neurological observations

Reason for undertaking GCS (circle)	Date started:
Fall with head injury / suspected head injury	Head injury
Encephalopathy	Seizure
CNS infection	Other (specify)

Frequency of neuro obs (circle):	half hour	every hour	every 2 hours	every 4 hours (see NICE for head injury)
Neuro obs to continue for (circle):	next 12 hours	24 hours	48 hours	72 hours
Revise EWS (circle):	Yes	No	If Yes trigger new threshold+	

Please enter date and time in boxes below

Date																										
Time																										

Glasgow Coma Scale

Eye opening

Spontaneous	4	4	4	4	4	4	4	4	4	4	4	4	4	4	4	4	4	4	4	4	4	4	4	Please circle appropriate score
To speech	3	3	3	3	3	3	3	3	3	3	3	3	3	3	3	3	3	3	3	3	3	3	3	
To pain	2	2	2	2	2	2	2	2	2	2	2	2	2	2	2	2	2	2	2	2	2	2	2	
None	1	1	1	1	1	1	1	1	1	1	1	1	1	1	1	1	1	1	1	1	1	1	1	

Motor response

Obeys commands	6	6	6	6	6	6	6	6	6	6	6	6	6	6	6	6	6	6	6	6	6	6	6	
Localises to pain	5	5	5	5	5	5	5	5	5	5	5	5	5	5	5	5	5	5	5	5	5	5	5	
Flexion	4	4	4	4	4	4	4	4	4	4	4	4	4	4	4	4	4	4	4	4	4	4	4	Any decrease in motor response add 4 to EWS
Abnormal flexion	3	3	3	3	3	3	3	3	3	3	3	3	3	3	3	3	3	3	3	3	3	3	3	
Extension	2	2	2	2	2	2	2	2	2	2	2	2	2	2	2	2	2	2	2	2	2	2	2	
None	1	1	1	1	1	1	1	1	1	1	1	1	1	1	1	1	1	1	1	1	1	1	1	

Verbal response

Orientated	5	5	5	5	5	5	5	5	5	5	5	5	5	5	5	5	5	5	5	5	5	5	5	
Confused	4	4	4	4	4	4	4	4	4	4	4	4	4	4	4	4	4	4	4	4	4	4	4	
Inappropriate	3	3	3	3	3	3	3	3	3	3	3	3	3	3	3	3	3	3	3	3	3	3	3	
Sounds	2	2	2	2	2	2	2	2	2	2	2	2	2	2	2	2	2	2	2	2	2	2	2	
None	1	1	1	1	1	1	1	1	1	1	1	1	1	1	1	1	1	1	1	1	1	1	1	

Totals																								

Limb movement

Arms

Normal power	
Mild weakness	
Severe weakness	
Spastic flexion	
Extension	
No response	

Legs

Normal power	
Mild weakness	
Severe weakness	
Spastic flexion	
Extension	
No response	

Place a cross in the box according to limb movement. Record right (R) and left (L) where the two sides are not the same.

Pupils

Pupils scale (mm)		
Right pupil size		
Right pupil		
Left pupil size		
Left pupil reaction		
Unequal		

+ Reacts
- No reaction
C Eyes closed
SL Sluggish

Total EWS (BOC + Neuro chart)		

Total EWS Score

Signature

ACTIONS if Neurological examination abnormal

If decrease in Motor score - add 4 to EWS score and call 6999 for urgent review.

If total GCS drops by 2 points or more - add 4 points to EWS score and call 6999 for urgent review

If total GCS drops by 1 point or more - add 2 points to EWS score. Patient must be reviewed by Nurse in charge and have a medical review.

Any unilateral pupil changes - add 4 to EWS score and call 6999 for urgent review.

Any new limb weakness - add 2 points to EWS score and patient must be reviewed by Nurse in charge and have medical review.

* If head injury suspected, patient requires neurological observations: half hourly for first two hours, hourly for next 4 hours and then 2 hourly if no change.

Figure 10.1 A neurological observation chart. Permission to reproduce this image is granted by North Bristol NHS Trust and University Hospitals Bristol NHS Foundation Trust

- *Score 4* if the patient withdraws from pain. This means that the patient flexes or bends the arm towards the source of pain, but fails to locate the source of pain (no wrist rotation).
- *Score 3* if the patient flexes to pain. This means that the patient flexes or bends the arm: this is characterised by internal rotation. Appears slower than normal flexion.
- *Score 2* if the patient shows extension to pain. This means that the patient extends the arm by straightening the elbow and possibly wrist rotation.
- *Score 1* if there is no response to painful stimuli.

Pupillary Assessment

This is conducted by observing the pre-assessment size and shape of the pupils and documenting it (in millimetres). The procedure is then conducted, as follows.

1 Wash your hands.
2 Explain the procedure to the patient (even if unconscious).
3 Dim the overhead lighting, if possible.
4 Move a torchlight from side of head towards the pupil and note any change in pupil size and speed of reaction (brisk or sluggish).
5 Check for consensual reflex (opposite pupil reaction).
6 Repeat the procedure in the opposite eye.
7 Document.

Patient may require a painful stimulus, whereby we would record that the patient is opening their eyes to pain, thus scoring 2 on the chart.

The Other Ds

After we have conducted the neurological assessments we also need to look at the other components of the D assessment; that is, *diabetes*, *drugs* and *diuresis*.

First we simply conduct a blood glucose test, as the blood glucose level may be a factor in why our patient is deteriorating, even if they are not known to have diabetes. We also look at the drug chart to see if there are any items with a bearing on our patient's condition, and seek to establish whether any drugs have been taken.

Now we come to the *diuresis* component. This assessment can be conducted by looking at the patient's fluid chart to check urine output, but this can only be done if they are actually having their fluids documented.

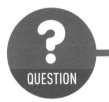

QUESTION

Question 10.1   What do these terms oliguria, anuria and absolute anuria mean?

We would look at our patient's condition as a whole to establish whether the kidneys were being fully perfused, as we know that conditions such as hypovolaemia, hypotension and dehydration would cause ineffective perfusion of the kidneys and have a direct bearing on the urine output. Renal perfusion requires 25% of cardiac output, so if our patient had experienced a recent cardiac assault the renal system would be directly affected. We could also look at our patient's prescription chart, as we know that certain drugs are nephrotoxic; that is, associated with structural damage to the nephrons in the kidneys. Some of these drugs include:

- *cardiac drugs*: angiotensin-converting enzyme (ACE) inhibitors, beta-blockers, radiocontrast media;
- *non-steroidal anti-inflammatory drugs*: diclofenac, ibuprofen;
- *antibiotics*: acyclovir, vancomycin, rifampicin, sulphonamides, ciprofloxacin;
- *diuretics*: furosemide.

If the disability assessment (neurological, blood glucose, diuresis and drugs) has not triggered action based on the EWS score, or any other concerns, we can move on to the exposure part of the assessment chain.

Exposure

This is where we literally expose our patient to observe wound sites, etc. The exposure assessment consists of looking for:

- blood or fluid loss,
- injuries or foreign objects,
- scars: surgical or other,
- skin colour: capillary refill,
- peripheral skin temperature,
- distal pulses: femoral/pedal,
- oedema.

We also check the patient's temperature and look at their observations and notes.

Remember Sandra Singh in Activity 10.1? Only when we pulled back her bed clothes did we notice she was bleeding profusely from her wound site and had actually gone into hypovolaemic shock.

This is how we conduct our ABCDE assessment, which is used in conjunction with EWS and SBAR, to recognise any deterioration in our patients. It allows us to act quickly and efficiently in providing care to reverse the situation, if possible.

TEST YOUR KNOWLEDGE

1 What does SBAR mean?
2 What does EWS mean?
3 What are the components of the ABCDE assessment?

KEY POINTS

- The SBAR communication tool.
- The Early Warning Score (EWS) system.
- Early Patient Assessment and Response (EPAR).

Chapter 11

INTRAVENOUS THERAPY

Clinical Skills for Nurses, First Edition. Claire Boyd
© 2013 John Wiley & Sons, Ltd. Published 2013 by John Wiley & Sons Ltd.

LEARNING OUTCOMES

By the end of this chapter you will have an understanding of the theory and practice of performing the clinical skill of intravenous therapy.

The general pubic expects to receive the right drug at the right time under the right conditions and the Government expects nothing less from National Health Service employees as part of clinical effectiveness. (Armitage and Knapman 2003)

It is now recognised practice that any qualified nursing, midwifery, radiography, registered operating department and anaesthetic practitioners, and assistant practitioners, who administer intravenous (IV) drugs must undertake a training programme, including an IV calculations test, and be assessed as competent to carry out this skill. In hospital environments all IV drugs must be second-checked by a qualified member of staff. In community settings this is not always possible and so extra care must be taken.

The above quote is not intended to scare you, just to make you think very carefully about IV therapy and to highlight the fact that if you are not careful and vigilant then accidents and incidents can, and do, occur.

POSSIBLE COMPLICATIONS

The possible complications of IV therapy include:

- cannula occlusion/damage,
- pain,
- phlebitis,
- embolism,
- drug error,
- needlestick injury,

- speed shock/fluid overload/free flow,
- extravasation,
- infiltration,
- haematoma.

We shall look at these complications individually.

Cannula Occlusion/Damage

We must never ignore a cannula occlusion as immediate action will be required.

A patient having IV drugs must have an access port *in situ*, usually a peripheral venous catheter (PVC) (see Chapter 9). The first thing we may notice with an occluded cannula is difficulty flushing the actual device. The patient may express pain at the cannula site, warranting an immediate resiting of a new cannula. If a patient is having IV fluids delivered via a pump then the pump alarms may be triggered. *Never ignore a pump alarm*: it will be sounding for a reason.

If the IV therapy was being administered without a pump – known as gravity feed – you may notice that the infusion has run very slowly, or even stopped at times.

When flushing a cannula you must use the push/pause technique with a 10 mL syringe or larger: nothing smaller than a 10 mL syringe should be used (see Chapter 9). Never force a flush because it may cause a clot at the end of the PVC to be dislodged, which would lead to a thrombotic event.

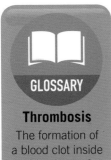

GLOSSARY

Thrombosis
The formation of a blood clot inside a blood vessel, obstructing the flow of blood through the circulatory system.

Pain

The cannula site should be inspected using the VIP score (meaning visual inspection of phlebitis; see Chapter 9). It should be remembered, however, that the patient's arm does not have to *look* painful to actually *be* painful.

Sometimes a cannula may have been sited in a poor position, such as over a joint, so that every time the joint is moved it causes pain. The cannula might also have become damaged.

A painful cannula site may also be due to the drug, perhaps if the wrong dilution has been used. Phenytoin has the same pH as bleach and can be very painful if a large cannula has been sited and, possibly, migrated out of the vein. The drug then starts to cause extravasation, eating away at the surrounding tissues.

Above all, *listen to the patient*.

Phlebitis may also be a cause of pain, and regular inspections should be made of the PVC device (see Chapter 9).

Embolism

There are three types of embolism, as follows.

- *Thrombus (blood clot)*: this is usually treated with oral anticoagulants, in most cases with drugs such as warfarin. Daily or alternate-day International Normalised Ratios (INRs) will need to be obtained.
- *Air* entering cardiovascular system, which is why we exclude air from IV administration sets and syringes. It does not take very much air in the system to cause death, probably as little as 8–10 mL.
- *Mechanical*: this is caused by a broken piece of cannula, glass from an ampoule or rubber from an ampoule getting into the system. Studies have shown that 50% of glass ampoules have glass shards at the bottom following their being snapped open. This is why it is so important to change needles after the medication has been drawn up, before the injection. Also, you must always check the cannula that you have removed. If you suspect that part of the tubing is missing the patient will require an X-ray to locate the missing section, which will have to be removed surgically.

Drug Errors

More patients are requiring IV therapy today than ever before, so we need to be expert when administering medication via this route (as with all medications, via all routes). However, up to 50% of all IV therapy drug administrations include a calculations error.

Activity 11.1

A patient is receiving IV therapy (1 L of sodium chloride 0.9%) for rehydration. The bag of fluid is prescribed to run over 8 hours. What is the drip rate per minute?

We notice that the patient has had 600 mL of the bag after just 4 hours. What is the revised drip rate to get this therapy back on track?

What actions would you take?

For drug errors involving infusions, we would need to stop running the infusion immediately and inform senior staff, including the nurse in charge, medic and pharmacist. We should always inform our patients of drug-related mistakes and offer reassurance and undertake relevant observations. Documentation will need to be completed. Nurses must be honest because the NHS is striving to learn from the mistakes in a 'non-blame culture', and to facilitate transparency in order for patients to have renewed faith in their NHS.

Needlestick Injury

- Needlestick injuries are most often caused by re-sheathing needles: never re-sheath a needle.
- Data suggests that most injuries occur after the procedure: so, put sharps straight into the sharps bin.
- Do not overfill sharps bins: they should only ever be three-quarters full or filled to the line markings before being sealed shut.
- Be careful when handling sharps: gloves will help to wipe off any of the patient's blood from a needle, minimising the amount of blood taken into your system.
- You should not use pulp trays, only clean rigid injection trays. Pulp trays are made from paper-mache and when the trays are wet sharps can penetrate this material.

- Read your local sharps handling policy and know what to do if you are injured.

If you have a needlestick injury, *administer first aid*:

- encourage the wound to bleed by squeezing,
- wash it thoroughly with running water,
- cover the wound with waterproof dressing,
- inform the nurse in charge and contact your local needlestick injury hotline and/or occupational health. Complete the necessary documentation.

Speed Shock/Fluid Overload/Free Flow

Speed shock is the rapid, uncontrolled administration of a drug, where symptoms occur as a result of the speed with which the medication is administered rather than the volume of drug or fluid. It can therefore occur even with small volumes. An example of this is a drug called furosemide which, if administered too fast, can cause tinnitus or permanent deafness. This drug has to be administered at a rate of 4 mg/minute.

Activity 11.2

ACTIVITY

A child has been prescribed 20 mg of furosemide daily. Over what time period should this bolus injection be administered?

When we add drugs to bags of fluids, we need to invert the bag several times to mix the mixture well. Otherwise, all the medication can fall to the bottom of the bag and be administered to the patient in far too concentrated a dose (what if the drug was potassium? We could have a fatality on our hands.).

Fluid overload is literally when we overload our patients with fluids: such as the patient in Activity 11.1. This can be very dangerous in 'at-risk' patients, such as cardiac patients, renal patients, older patients and children.

Free flow is when the fluid we are administering is not regulated. Fluid overload can result from this.

Dougherty (2011) sums up this well:

> ...the administration of medication and/or infusion should be performed over the specified time in order to prevent the development of speed shock and fluid overload.

The causes and complications of free flow are:

- potentially very dangerous,
- if patient is at risk, i.e. with cardiac failure, avoid free flow by using a pump,
- if using a gravity feed remember your drip rate formula,
- observe infusion frequently,
- beware if the cannula is 'positional'; that is, improperly sited in the vein and prone to being dislodged,
- confused patients may open a clamp or valve,
- inform medical staff immediately if free flow has occurred. Perform accurate vital sign monitoring. Document all incidents.

Extravasation

This is when a vesicant (blister-forming) substance eats away at the underlying tissue due to a cannula coming out of a vein (see also Chapter 9). It takes very little time for this to occur. Treatment is usually for adrenaline to be injected into the surrounding area and for saline or water flushes to dilute the drug in the patient's tissues. Also, as much of the drug as possible may be drawn out using a needle and syringe. Ice is applied to the damaged area and analgesia prescribed to ease the patient's pain.

Many oncology drugs may cause extravasation, and children are particularly prone because they have smaller veins. Extravasation can therefore occur more frequently in these clinical areas.

Infiltration

This used to be referred to as 'tissuing'. Infiltration occurs when a cannula dislodges from the vein and the infused substance runs into the tissues. The arm can become oedematous (very swollen). Treatment is usually by raising the patient's arm so that the infusion may be absorbed slowly into the bodily tissues.

We know that infiltration can cause permanent nerve damage and a patient may require an escharotomy, surgery to 'spilt and drain' to remove this excess fluid. As little as 500 mL of fluid can cause permanent nerve damage.

Haematoma

Haematomas are caused by uncontrollable bleeding, usually creating a hard, discoloured, painful swelling under the skin.

PROCEDURE FOR THE ADMINISTRATION OF IV FLUIDS VIA GRAVITY

1	Collect all equipment.
2	Wash your hands.
3	Gloves must be worn if giving antibiotic therapy (sterile gloves are not required). Two checkers are required for IV therapy.
4	Apply aseptic principles.
5	Check that you are with the correct patient and gain consent.
6	Inspect the fluid bag to be certain that it contains the correct fluid, the fluid is clear (if the medication should be), the bag is not leaking and the bag has not expired.
7	Sterile packaging must not be damaged or wet.
8	Ensure that you have the correct giving set for the fluid to be administered, as different sets are required for blood and blood products and for electronic devices. These sets are either microdrip sets, which deliver 60 drops per ml into the drip chamber, or macrodrip sets, which deliver 15–20 drops per ml into the drip chamber.

9	Open the packaging and uncoil the tubing: do not let the ends of the tubing become contaminated. Close the flow regulator (roll the wheel away from the end to which you will attach the fluid bag).
10	Remove the protective covering from the port of the fluid bag and the protective covering from the spike of the administration set.
11	Insert the spike of the administration set into the port of the fluid bag with a quick twist. Do this carefully. Be especially careful not to puncture yourself! Insert this spike fully into the infusion bag, as this is an infection risk.
12	Hold the fluid bag higher than the drip chamber of the administration set. Squeeze the drip chamber once or twice to start the flow. Fill the drip chamber to one-third full. If you overfill the chamber, lower the bag below the level of the drip chamber and squeeze some fluid back into the fluid bag.
13	Open the flow regulator and allow the fluid to flush all the air from the tubing. Let it run into the giving set's empty packaging or container. You may need to loosen or remove the cap at the end of the tubing to get the fluid to flow to the end of the tubing (but this should not be necessary), taking care not to let the tip of the administration set become contaminated.
14	The primed giving set is now ready to be connected to a electronic device, or the rate can be determined by gravity flow together with the flow clamp.
15	Connect the end of the tubing to the patient: the IV cannula must be of an appropriate size for the intended use and cleaned before the administration set line end is attached, to minimise infection risk.
16	Document the procedure and initiate a fluid chart document.

TEST YOUR KNOWLEDGE

This is a scenario exercise. You may wish to see if you can borrow copy of the *British National Formulary* (BNF) for this exercise or just have a go at answering as much as you can.

Mrs Jones is admitted to hospital with a systemic bacterial infection, thought to be respiratory in origin. She has been prescribed Flagyl 500 mg QDS and Cefuroxime 750 mg QDS. You are a third-year student nurse, on your last placement. The nurse you are working with is a registered general nurse (RGN) and very experienced at administering IV medication.

The RGN mixes the two antibiotics together, ready for the midnight dose. You are asked to check the medication. You assume the two antibiotics can be mixed, as this nurse is very experienced. You check the medication and all seems fine, all is in date and prescribed for the right patient. You go through the checks:

- right medicine,
- right dose,
- right route,
- right patient,
- right time.

The experienced nurse checks the patient's identity bands to check the patient and administers the medication without any problems and disposes of the sharps correctly. The drug chart is signed appropriately.

At 02:30 the patient complains of feeling nauseous and has developed diarrhoea. She states she feels very unwell. The clinical site manager (CSM) is paged and shortly arrives on the ward. The CSM looks at the drug chart and at once notices the mistake.

1 What mistakes have been made?
2 What actions should be taken?

KEY POINTS

- **Possible complications of IV therapy.**
- **Procedure for the administration of IV fluids via the gravity procedure.**

Chapter 12
BASIC LIFE SUPPORT

Clinical Skills for Nurses, First Edition. Claire Boyd

LEARNING OUTCOMES

By the end of this chapter you will have an understanding of the theory and practice of providing basic life support.

Cardiopulmonary arrest can occur at any time and in any place and you will be given training in basic life support during your mandatory and statutory training programme in your corporate induction to the work environment. You will learn during these sessions about the recovery position and jaw thrust, chin lift and how to use a 'stand back!' automated external defibrillator (AED).

The Resuscitation Council (UK) states that the difference between basic life support and advanced life support is 'arbitrary', as in the hospital setting these processes are on a continuum.

This chapter is a guide to in-hospital adult and paediatric basic life support, based on the document *2010 International Consensus on Cardiopulmonary Resuscitation and Emergency Cardiovascular Care Science with Treatment Recommendations* (Nolan et al., 2010), published in October 2010. It is aimed at healthcare professionals who are first to respond to an in-hospital cardiac arrest.

In the acute hospital environment many areas have four cardiac arrest teams that respond to emergency calls:

- adult,
- paediatric (children less than 16 years of age),
- maternal (pregnant women),
- neonatal.

You will need to know how to summon emergency assistance in your area; that is, what the call number is (often 2222) and the line of order (team dynamics) within the emergency responders. You should also familiarise yourself with the resuscitation trolley, perhaps by getting involved in the daily or weekly checks of this equipment, and the emergency drug box. You should certainly be aware of where to find the defibrillator and all the emergency equipment, as it may be you who is asked to be the 'runner' who collects anything required by the emergency team.

Those in community settings, without a cardiac arrest team, will often need to dial 999 for an ambulance, detailing the nature of the incident and performing basic life support until help arrives.

Whichever setting you work in, you need to be aware of whether a patient has legal documentation stating 'do not attempt cardiopulmonary resuscitation' in their medical notes. It is ultimately the consultant's responsibility to arrange this legal notice. Other documentation to be aware of is the paperwork recorded after an in-hospital event. This is part of the standardised data collected by the National Cardiac Arrest Audit as part of an audit and quality-improvement process.

After any emergency event, such as a cardiac arrest, it is good practice for staff to debrief. This will give everyone a chance to state what went well with the procedure and what did not go quite so well; this feedback is vital to improve everyone's performance in emergency events.

Patients who witnessed the flurry of activity surrounding an emergency event may be quite distressed, so some kind words, reassurance and perhaps a cup of tea will go a long way towards settling them.

The Resuscitation Council (UK) states that we must ensure three things.

1   The cardiorespiratory arrest is recognised immediately.
2   Help is summoned.
3   Cardiopulmonary resuscitation (CPR) is started immediately and, if indicated, defibrillation is attempted immediately (within 3 minutes).

RESPONDING TO AN EMERGENCY EVENT

The Collapsed Adult Patient

- On finding our collapsed patient, or witnessing a collapse, we must first ensure our own personal safety and then immediately shout for help.
- Then we need to check the patient for a response. This is done by gently shaking their shoulders and asking loudly 'Are you alright?'

The Responsive Patient

- If the patient responds, obtain an urgent medical assessment: this may be from the resuscitation team.
- While waiting for the medical assessment, administer oxygen therapy and assess the patient using the ABCDE approach and attach monitoring to record vital signs; for example, pulse oximetry, ECG, blood pressure, etc. (see Chapter 10).
- Obtain venous access.
- Hand over to the team using the SBAR communication tool (see Chapter 10).

This is the in-hospital resuscitation algorithm for the responsive patient:

- collapsed/sick patient,
- shout for HELP and assess patient,
- signs of Life? Yes,
- assess ABCDE,
- recognise and treat. Oxygen, monitoring, IV access,
- call resuscitation team, if appropriate,
- hand over to resuscitation team.

The Unresponsive Patient

- Shout for help again (if this has not already been obtained).
- Turn the patient on their back and open the airway using the head tilt and chin-lift technique. If you suspect

a cervical spine injury then use only the jaw thrust to open the airway. An airway adjunct may be inserted.

- Quickly: listen, look and feel to determine whether the patient is breathing normally. This is performed by *listening* at the victim's mouth for breath sounds, *looking* for chest movement and *feeling* for air on your cheek.
- Listen for agonal breathing: this is when we hear occasional gasps, and slow, laboured or noisy breathing, and is common immediately after a cardiac arrest and should not be taken as a sign of life.
- More experienced staff may feel for a carotid pulse.

The Patient Has a Pulse or Other Signs of Life

- Urgent medical assessment is required. While waiting for the assessment, administer oxygen therapy and assess the patient using the ABCDE approach and attach monitoring to record vital signs; for example, pulse oximetry, ECG, blood pressure, etc. (see Chapter 10).
- Obtain venous access.
- Hand over to the team using the SBAR communication tool (see Chapter 10).

The Patient Does Not Have a Pulse or Other Signs of Life

- One person starts CPR, one person calls the resuscitation team and one person collects the resuscitation equipment and a defibrillator. If only one person is present at this time, this will mean leaving the patient.
- Give *30 chest compressions followed by two ventilations*.
- The correct hand position for chest compressions is the middle of the lower half of the sternum and the depth of the compressions should be 5–6 cm at a rate of at least 100 compressions each minute (but no more than 120). The chest should recoil completely between each compression.

- The person providing chest compressions should change every 2 minutes, so as not to fatigue. This switch should be conducted with the minimum amount of disruption to compressions.
- The airway should be maintained and the lungs ventilated. An airway adjunct may be placed *in situ* and a bag mask may be used for this ventilation, according to local policy, with supplemental oxygen therapy. If mouth-to-mouth ventilation is not commencing, continue with chest compressions until help or airway equipment arrives.
- When the defibrillator arrives, apply the self-adhesive pads to the patient, while still continuing with the chest compressions. Only those trained to use the defibrillator may use these machines and defibrillate if appropriate.
- Advanced life support: when resuscitation team arrive. Hand over to the resuscitation team leader using the SBAR communication tool.
- Once sufficient staff are present you may be required to prepare intravenous cannulation and/or any drugs required by the resuscitation team.

This is the in-hospital resuscitation algorithm for the unresponsive patient:

- collapsed/sick patient,
- shout for HELP and assess patient,
- signs of life? No,
- call resuscitation team,
- CPR compression/ventilation ratio 30:2 with oxygen and airway adjuncts,
- apply pads/monitor. Attempt defibrillation if appropriate,
- advanced life support when resuscitation team arrives.

Respiratory Arrest: if the Patient is Not Breathing but has a Pulse

- Ventilate the patient's lungs and check for a pulse every 10 breaths. Only those competent in assessing breathing and a pulse will be able to make the diagnosis of respiratory arrest, so start chest compressions if there is any doubt about the presence of a pulse. Continue until more experienced help arrives.

THE PHONETIC ALPHABET

We have already discussed the SBAR communication tool, but during fraught moments our verbalisation may become a little garbled. When we put out an emergency call we need to have complete clarity in informing the emergency team of the exact location of the event. To do this, we might use the phonetic alphabet. For example, we may need the resuscitation team to come to 'D for Delta Ward'.

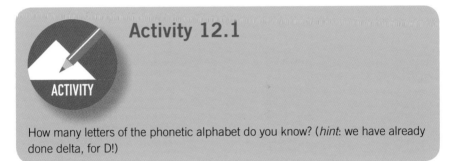

Activity 12.1

ACTIVITY

How many letters of the phonetic alphabet do you know? (*hint*: we have already done delta, for D!)

PAEDIATRIC BASIC LIFE SUPPORT

The Resuscitation Council (UK) states that many children receive no resuscitation due to the fact that many rescuers fear that they will cause harm as they have received no paediatric resuscitation training. However, research tells us that performing either chest compressions or expired air ventilation may result in a better outcome than doing nothing at all. Arrests of cardiac origin are seen predominantly in adults, while it is the asphyxial arrests that occur more commonly in children. Therefore a separate paediatric algorithm has been devised of two rescue breaths and 15 compressions (but starting with five rescue breaths), giving us a CPR compression/ventilation ratio of

2:15. Chest-compression depths are at 4 cm for infants and 5 cm for children, with the rate being the same as for adult basic life support: 100 compressions per minute, but not greater than 120 per minute. The recommended compression/ventilation ratio for newborn babies is 3:1.

This is the algorithm for paediatric basic life support:

- unresponsive?
- shout for help,
- open airway,
- not breathing normally?
- five rescue breaths,
- no sign of life?
- 15 chest compressions,
- CPR compression/ventilation ratio: two rescue breaths to 15 compressions,
- call resuscitation team.

TEST YOUR KNOWLEDGE

1 What is the chest compression/ventilation ratio for an adult?
2 At what depth should these compressions be?
3 What is the chest compression/ventilation ratio for an infant?
4 At what depth should these compressions be?
5 At what rate should the compressions be given for an adult?
6 At what rate should the compressions be given for a child?
7 In the phonetic alphabet, what word represents K?

KEY POINTS

- Adult basic life support.
- The phonetic alphabet.
- Paediatric basic life support.

Answers to Activities, Questions and "Test Your Knowledge"

CHAPTER 1

Activity 1.1

Did you notice that it is only the systolic blood pressure recording that generates a score on the chart in the blood pressure section? So, only the blood pressure of 202 mmHg generated a score, of 2.

Activity 1.2

102 bpm generates a score of 1.

Activity 1.3

Cyanosis	Cyanosed/blue tinge to skin, lips, nail beds or in the mucous membrane (in mouth). Anaemic patients may have insufficient haemoglobin to produce cyanotic appearance.
Blood gases	Increased carbon dioxide make the blood values acidic. Increased oxygen make the blood values alkaline. Normal values = pH 7.35–7.45. Respiratory acidosis occurs if pH is below 7.28 (likelihood of death).
Hypoxia	Lack of oxygen in the tissues.
Hypercapnia	Higher than normal levels of carbon dioxide in the bodily tissues.
Hypoxaemia	Decreased oxygen levels in arterial blood.
Tidal volume	The amount of air breathed in and out during a single breath (normally 500 mL).
Total lung capacity	The amount of air the lungs can hold: approximately 5 L.
Residual volume	The volume of air remaining in the lungs at the end of a forceful expiration.

Chapter 1 Questions

1.1 (1) To establish a baseline reading; (2) to monitor fluctuations in temperature, i.e. fever, ovulation in women; (3) to monitor signs

Clinical Skills for Nurses, First Edition. Claire Boyd
© 2013 John Wiley & Sons, Ltd. Published 2013 by John Wiley & Sons Ltd.

of incompatibility during blood transfusion; (4) to monitor the temperature of patients being treated for infection; (5) to monitor the temperature of patients recovering from hypothermia.

1.2 Temporal, carotid, brachial, radial, femoral, popliteal, posterior tibial, dorsalis pedis

Chapter 1 Test Your Knowledge

EWS values: respiratory rate, 1; SpO$_2$, 0; blood pressure, 0; heart rate, 2; neurological response (AVPU), 0; temperature, 1; total EWS, 4. Action: re-check score. Inform nurse in charge. Request a medical review within 15 minutes. Record the action taken and the result of the medical review.

CHAPTER 2

Activity 2.1

Chapter 2 Questions

2.1 A urethral stricture is damage to the urethral lining.

2.2 A priapism is a persistent and often painful erection that requires immediate decompression. It may be caused by local or spinal cord damage.

Chapter 2 Test Your Knowledge

1 Clean intermittent (CIC), urethral (URC), suprapubic (SPC) catheterisation.

2 CIC: can give individuals independence and control over their own bodies; URC, suitable for most patients requiring bladder drainage; SPC, can be used if URC is unsuitable (i.e. due to trauma).

3 CIC, patients must have good dexterity and cognitive function to be able to self-care; URC, high risk of infection (CAUTI);

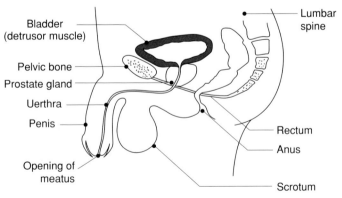

Bladder (detrusor muscle)
Pelvic bone
Prostate gland
Uerthra
Penis
Opening of meatus
Lumbar spine
Rectum
Anus
Scrotum

Permission to reproduce this image is granted by North Bristol NHS Trust and University Hospitals Bristol NHS Foundation Trust

SPC, contra-indicated in bladder tumours or unexplained haematuria.

4 Urethral trauma resulting in infection and possible septicaemia/renal failure/death; formation of false urethral passage; bladder perforation; traumatic removal of catheter with balloon inflated; UTI and possible septicaemia/renal failure/death; by-passing of urine around catheter. Also, urethral stricture formation, meatal tears, encrustation and bladder calculi, urethral perforation, pain, bleeding, bladder spasm, reduced bladder capacity, catheter blockage, latex sensitivity, altered body image, difficulties with sexual relations.

5 Within 48 hours of prostate surgery; history of urethral stricture; history of bacteraemia associated with catheterisation unless patient has been given appropriate prophylaxis (discuss with microbiologist); priapism (a persistent and usually painful erection of the penis that requires urgent decompression).

6 Catheter valve: every 7 days; catheter drainage bags: 7 days; catheter 'belly bags': every 28 days.

7 Talcum powder and creams must not be used around catheter sites.

8 Catheter type, length and size; batch number; manufacturer; amount of water instilled into the balloon; date and time of catheterisation; reasons for catheterisation; colour of urine drained; any problems negotiated during the procedure; a review date to assess the need for continued catheterisation, or date of change of catheter.

9 From the sample port on the drainage bag. The port must be cleaned prior to the procedure. Urine samples must never be taken by emptying the bag via the drainage tap.

10 After emptying catheter bag the port should be decontaminated with alcohol wipes.

CHAPTER 3

Activity 3.1

See figure on top of the next page.

Chapter 3 Questions

3.1 If you take out the catheter tube, subsequent tubes may follow the same tract into the vagina. By leaving the tube in place, we will hopefully avoid this wrong tract a second time.

Chapter 3 Test Your Knowledge

1 Gain consent.

2 From the pubic bone at the front to the bottom of the backbone.

3 Soap and water.

4 For the same reasons as male catheterisation: for drainage, investigation and instillation purposes. It may also be performed during childbirth.

Activity 3.1

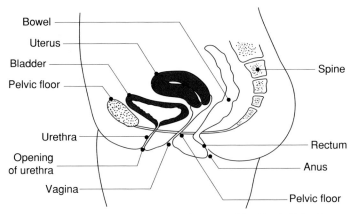

Bowel
Uterus
Bladder
Pelvic floor
Spine
Urethra
Rectum
Opening of urethra
Anus
Vagina
Pelvic floor

Permission to reproduce this image is granted by North Bristol NHS Trust and University Hospitals Bristol NHS Foundation Trust

CHAPTER 4

Chapter 4 Questions

4.1 (1) Storage: the colon stores unabsorbed food residue. Within 72 hours of intake 70% of food residue has been excreted. The remaining 30% stays in the colon for up to a week. The longer food residue remains in the colon, the more water is absorbed and the harder the stools that are produced. (2) Absorption: sodium, water, chloride and some fat-soluble vitamins are all absorbed from the colon. Some drugs, for example some steroids and aspirin, are also absorbed by the colon. (3) Secretion: mucus is secreted by the colon to lubricate the faeces and aid expulsion. (4) Synthesis of some vitamins: bacteria which colonize the colon are responsible for the production of small amounts of vitamin K, thiamine, folic acid and riboflavin. (5) Elimination: the main function of the colon is the absorption of fluid and the peristaltic movement of faecal matter into the rectum, which has sensory nerve endings that generate the sensation of fullness, followed by a desire to defecate.

4.2 Impaction with faecal overflow, pelvic floor damage, neurological disease (such as cerebral disease, spinal cord problems), colon disorders (such as carcinoma, colitis, diverticulitis, irritable bowel syndrome), surgical trauma, diarrhoea (caused by infections such as gastroenteritis), endocrine disorders (such as diabetes).

Chapter 4 Test Your Knowledge

1 Storage, absorption, secretion, synthesis of some vitamins, elimination
2 The Bristol Stool Chart
3 Digital rectal examination
4 Autonomic dysreflexia
5 Distended bladder (e.g. catheter blockage or bladder outlet obstruction), distended bowel (e.g. constipation or impaction or full rectum), ingrown toenail, fracture below level of the lesion, pressure ulcer, contact burn, scald or sunburn, urinary tract infections or bladder spasms, renal or bladder calculi, pain or trauma, deep vein thrombosis, over-stimulation during sexual activity, severe anxiety
6 To trigger reflex relaxation of internal sphincter and promote emptying of the rectum.

CHAPTER 5

Chapter 5 Test Your Knowledge

1 Tenacious: holding or sticking firmly. In other words, thick sticky secretions. Would be treated with nebulisation to thin the secretions to make them easier to remove by suction.
2 Bifurcating: a point at which division of two branches occurs, such as in the bronchial tree descending into the lungs.

3 Kyphoscoliosis: kyphosis combined with scoliosis. Abnormal curvature of the spine both forwards and sideways.
4 INR: International Normalized Ratio, or INR, is a measurement of blood clotting time. The higher the INR, the longer it will take for your blood to clot (see Chapter 8 for more details).

CHAPTER 6

Activity 6.1

1 pH 4.5–8.0
2 Diabetic ketoacidosis, starvation, potassium depletion, high-protein diet
3 The formation of renal calculi (stones)
4 Urinary tract infection (UTI), excessive vomiting, consumption of large amounts of antacids, diet high in vegetables, citrus fruits and dairy products
5 A stale urine specimen

Chapter 6 Test Your Knowledge

1 Urine pH, protein, glucose, ketones and blood
2 2 hours
3 Away from flammable substances and potential ignition sources
4 The upper outer aspects of the fingers or the outer heel for babys
5 Low blood sugar level

CHAPTER 7

Activity 7.1

Washed cells: here the plasma proteins are washed away from the plasma, leaving the cells only. This procedure is performed on blood for individuals who have previously reacted to a transfusion. This procedure is very expensive and performed by the National Blood Transfusion Service.

CMV: this is stands for cytomegalovirus, a type of herpes virus related to the cold sore, which many of us carry. In people with strong immune systems the virus remains inactive, but those with compromised immune systems need to have their transfused blood more finely filtered to remove any traces of the virus.

Irradiated blood: this is given to patients with conditions such as Hodgkin's disease and for babies *in utero*.

Activity 7.2

Registered or student nurse/midwife
    assistant practitioner and trainee
    assistant practitioner
Operating department practitioner/
    assistant
Healthcare assistant
Ward clerk/receptionist
Designated theatre porters

But only if trained to do so.

Activity 7.3

Red blood cells are stored in the fridge at 2–6°C. They must be returned to the fridge, and signed back in after 30 minutes if not going to be put up immediately. Platelets and FFP will not be stored in the fridge, but can be obtained from the laboratory. This is because platelets need to be kept moving as they want to do what comes naturally, which is clumping together to create a fibrin mesh. Clot formation is a safety measure to stop us from bleeding to death every time we have a cut. FFP is frozen to −30°C and needs to be thawed by the laboratory and then transfused immediately.

Chapter 7 Test Your Knowledge

1   Temperature, pulse, blood pressure and respiratory rate; these need to be done before collection, 15 minutes after transfusion starts and at the end of transfusion.

2   Temperature rises by 1°C.

CHAPTER 8

Chapter 8 Questions

8.1 (1) Obtaining blood to rule out conditions, such as obtaining electrolyte levels, e.g. sodium, potassium and urea. (2) To monitor levels of blood components, such as obtaining a full blood count to ascertain the number of red blood cells and their quality, and obtaining a cross-match prior to surgery. (3) Obtaining blood for diagnosis, such as cardiac enzymes, and liver function, e.g. enzymes released by the liver, and blood glucose readings. (4) To monitor blood levels, such as looking at levels of drugs in the blood, such as warfarin and phenytoin, which can be toxic.

8.2 List four of the tests described in the section Common Blood Tests.

Chapter 8 Test Your Knowledge

1 It is recommended that a tourniquet should not be left *in situ* for more than 1 minute; this also promotes patient comfort.

2 It has been shown to alter some blood results.

3 The blood sample tubes must be taken in that order, as recommended by the manufacturer or pathology laboratory.

4 Adults over 18 years are presumed able to give consent (with mental capacity).

5 Hepatitis B

6 Valid consent

7 Doctor, registered nurse or midwife trained in phlebotomy, phlebotomist, assistant practitioner or healthcare assistant trained in phlebotomy.

8 The time at which the last dose of the drug was taken.

CHAPTER 9

Chapter 9 Questions

9.1 (1) Fluid and electrolyte replacement; (2) intravenous drug therapy; (3) transfusions; (4) prophylaxis; (5) the administration of dyes and contrast media.

9.2

Extravasation	This is when a vesicant (blister-forming) substance eats away at the underlying tissue due to a cannula coming out of a vein.
Infiltration	This occurs when a cannula dislodges from a vein and the infused substance enters the surrounding tissues. The area can become oedematous (very swollen). It used to be referred to as 'tissuing'.

Chapter 9 Test Your Knowledge

1 Usually only immediately after the cannula has first been inserted.

2 The push/pause technique.

3 Always use the smallest possible cannula in the largest possible vein.

4 1.9. L/hour

5 Nothing smaller than a 10 mL syringe. Otherwise, too much pressure may be applied.

6 Visual inspection of phlebitis.

CHAPTER 10

Chapter 10 Questions

10.1

Oliguria	Production of abnormally small amounts of urine. May be caused by conditions such as excessive sweating, kidney disease, loss of blood or diarrhoea.
Anuria	This is when the kidneys fail to produce urine or the output is less than 100 mL in 24 hours.
Absolute anuria	Absence of urine output, generally reflecting a form of obstruction.

Activity 10.1

EWS values: respiratory rate, 1; SpO_2, 1; blood pressure, 1; heart rate, 2; neurological response (AVPU), 1; temperature, 0; total EWS, 6. Action: re-check score. Inform nurse in charge. Request a medical review within 15 minutes. Record the action taken and the result of the medical review.

Chapter 10 Test Your Knowledge

1 Situation, background, assessment, recommendation: a communication tool
2 Early Warning Score
3 Airway, breathing, circulation (cannulation), disability and diuresis (drugs and diabetes), exposure and early call for help using SBAR.

CHAPTER 11

Activity 11.1

We use the following formula, remembering that clear fluids are administered at 20 drops/mL:

$$Rate = \frac{volume}{time \ in \ hours} \times \frac{drops \ per \ millilitre}{60 \ minutes}$$

So:

$$\frac{1000 \ mL}{8 \ hours} \times \frac{20 \ drops/mL}{60 \ minutes}$$
$$= 42 \ drops \ per \ minute$$

Now we need to adjust the drip rate to get this medication back on track, using three steps.

1 How much of the bag is left?
1000 mL − 600 mL = 400 mL left
2 How much time is left? 8 hours − 4 hours = 4 hours left
3 Use the formula:

$$Rate = \frac{volume}{rate} \times \frac{drops \ per \ millilitre}{60 \ minutes}$$

$$\frac{400 \ mL}{42 \ drops/mL} \times \frac{20 \ drops/mL}{60 \ minutes}$$

$$= 3.17 \ drops \ per \ minute$$

So, we change the drip rate to approximately 3 drops per minute.

We would need to inform the patient that a drug error has occurred and complete all documentation in relation to this. A medic will also need to be informed.

Activity 11.2

This drug should be given:

$$\frac{Dose}{Rate} = \frac{20 \ mg}{4 \ mg/minute} = 5 \ minutes$$

Chapter 11 Test Your Knowledge

- Flagyl is a trade name and should have been prescribed as metronidazole.
- IV metronidazole should be prescribed every 8 hours, which is TDS and not QDS. The patient has been given the drug four times in 1 day instead of three times in 24 hours.
- Cefuroxime is prescribed as QDS: this is correct as this drug can be prescribed QDS or TDS; that is, every 6 or 8 hours.
- These two antibiotics can be mixed, but TDS drugs are usually given at 08:00, 16:00 and 24:00 and QDS drugs are usually given at 06:00, 12:00, 18:00 and 24:00, we can see only once in 24 hours can these drugs actually be given together. Also it is not a good idea to mix antibiotics because if the patient has a reaction we will not know which drug has caused the reaction.
- Side effects of metronidazole include gastrointestinal disturbances, such as nausea and vomiting: is our patient having a reaction to the medications, or an overdose of medication?
- Did anyone check whether Mrs Jones is allergic to antibiotics by asking her or checking her notes? Are we seeing the start of an anaphylaxis event?
- Just because the RGN was a very experienced nurse, did the student

not check all prescriptions herself? Why not?
- A student nurse without a PIN number (that's a nurse's unique identification number, issued by the Nursing and Midwifery Council) should not be a second checker. Student nurses can be a third checker only, because they have not yet been assessed for the administration of IV medications.
- Documentation should be completed following the drug error, but first the patient should be told of the error, and apologies given.
- A medic would need to be informed of the drug error.
- The patient would require close observation.

CHAPTER 12

Activity 12.1

Letter	Phonetic	Letter	Phonetic
A	Alpha	N	November
B	Bravo	O	Oscar
C	Charlie	P	Papa
D	Delta	Q	Quebec
E	Echo	R	Romeo
F	Foxtrot	S	Sierra
G	Golf	T	Tango
H	Hotel	U	Uniform
I	India	V	Victor
J	Juliet	W	Whiskey
K	Kilo	X	X-ray
L	Lima	Y	Yankee
M	Mike	Z	Zulu

Chapter 12 Test Your Knowledge

1 30:2
2 5–6 cm depth
3 15:2, but starting with five rescue breaths
4 4 cm
5 100 per minute (not greater than 120 per minute)
6 100 per minute (not greater than 120 per minute)
7 Kilo

Appendix 1

THE BRISTOL OBSERVATION CHART

Clinical Skills for Nurses, First Edition. Claire Boyd
© 2013 John Wiley & Sons, Ltd. Published 2013 by John Wiley & Sons Ltd.

Bristol Observation Chart

Hospital No.:				
Surname:				
Forename(s):				
Gender:		**D.o.B.:**		
Consultant:				

Date	/ /	/ /	/ /	/ /
Frequency of obs				

(eg. hourly, 4 hourly, 6 hourly BD, daily)

Ward:	Date																						
	Time																						
Resp. Rate	36+																						
	31-35																						
	26-30																						
	21-25																						
	15-20																						
	9-14																						
	≤8																						
SpO2	YES	Y	Y	Y	Y	Y	Y	Y	Y	Y	Y	Y	Y	Y	Y	Y	Y	Y	Y	Y	Y	Y	Y
Oxygen in prescribed range? Yes / No (see reverse)	93+																						
	90-92																						
	85-89																						
	<85																						
	NO	N	N	N	N	N	N	N	N	N	N	N	N	N	N	N	N	N	N	N	N	N	N
Delivered O2 (L/min/%)																							

Blood Pressure	200					
	190					
	180					
Record Systolic & Diastolic	170					
	160					
	150					
	140					
Score Systolic BP only	130					
	120					
	110					
	100					
	90					
	80					
	70					
	60					
	50					

Heart Rate	160		
	150		
	140		
	130		
	120		
	110		
	100		
	90		
	80		
	70		
	60		
	50		
	40		
	30		

Neuro Response	Alert
	Verbal
	Pain
	Unresp

Temp.	39°
	38°
	37°
	36°
	35°
	34°

EWS Score (score with all obs)	
Staff member (Initials) completing Obs.	

Patient not for score system		EWS Score:	☐ 0	☐ 1	2	3	Revised Trigger	
Initial (Cons. or SpR)							Initial (Cons. or SpR)	

Oxygen Administration

- Administer O$_2$ to achieve saturation in prescribed range.

- Only administer oxygen if it is prescribed - except in an emergency when oxygen may be given and actions recorded in medical notes later.

- **Increase** oxygen dose if saturation below range.

- **Decrease** oxygen dose or stop supplimentary oxygen if saturation exceeds target range. High levels of oxygen are harmful to some patients.

Target Oxygen Saturation Range

(Copy selected range from drug chart and circle).

94 - 98% (Age < 70yrs)	92 - 98% (Age > 70yrs)	88 - 92% (Risk factors present)

Prescription copied by: .... Date: ....

Patient not for O$_2$ monitoring ☐ | Reason

Patient not tolerating O$_2$ ☐

Signed: .... Date: ....

Action Report - EWS ≥4

Date	Time	Comment	Action Taken	Initials

(Brief report on response to EWS ≥4)

How to use the Bristol Observation Chart

Start up

1 Put patient identification label in top right hand corner.

2 Identify frequency for observations in the boxes provided.

3 If patient is not for EWS e.g. palliative care then Consultant or SpR to initial box on bottom right of chart.

4 In patients who are chronically unwell with physiological parameters that trigger EWS regularly a Consultant or SpR may decide to adjust trigger at which medical review is requested. This should be recorded in the appropriate box.

5 Copy target oxygen saturation range from drugs chart. If saturation range is changed start new chart.

Observations

1 Record ALL observations with a 'firm' dot ●

2 Join consecutive observations with a straight line.

3 Note whether observation falls in shaded 'at risk' zone. Score as per EWS key.

4 If observations lie on border betweeen EWS scores record **higher** score.

5 Check whether SpO$_2$ is in prescribed range (see below). Ring 'Y' (Yes) or 'N' (No). If No then inform nurse in charge immediately.

EWS scores

1 Total the EWS score using 0 to 3 scoring guide on the chart.

2 Record the total EWS score in the box for EWS.

☐ 0   ☐ 1

☐ 2   ▨ 3

EWS 0-1 : Routine observations

EWS 2-3 : Hourly observations and inform nurse in charge

EWS ≥4 : Inform nurse in charge and request medical review within 15 mins. **Complete report of action above**

Action

EWS SCORE 0 – 1

Continue with routine observations.

EWS SCORE 2-3

1 Inform nurse in charge.

2 Nurse to alter frequency of obs to e.g. hourly in box at top of chart

3 Record obs at new frequency.

EWS SCORE ≥4

1 Re-check score.

2 Inform nurse in charge.

3 Request medical review within 15 minutes.

4 Record action taken and result of medical review in box on reverse of obs. chart.

BOC V3 July 2010-07-15

Permission to reproduce this image is granted by North Bristol NHS Trust and University Hospitals Bristol NHS Foundation Trust.

Bibliography

Abd-el-Maeboud, K.H., el-Naggar, T., el-Hawi, E.M., Mahmoud, S.A. and Abd-el-Hay, S. (1991) Rectal suppository: common sense and mode of insertion. *The Lancet* 338 (8870), 798–800.

Anon (1999) Quick Reference Guide 8: Urine Testing. *Nursing Standard* 13(50).

Anon (2001) Essential skills: a monthly collectable guide to core clinical procedures. Observation and monitoring. 13. Recording temperature. *Nursing Standard* 15(38): insert 12.

Armitage, G. and Knapman, H. (2003) Adverse events in drug administration: a literature review. *Journal of Nursing Management* 11, 130–140.

Boyd, S., Aggarwal, I., Davey, P. et al. (2011) Peripheral intravenous catheters: the road to quality improvement and safer patient care. *Journal of Hospital Infection* 77, 37–41.

Brooks, D., Anderson, C.M., Carter, M.A. et al (2001) Clinical practice guidelines for suctioning the airway of the intubated and non-intubated patient. *Canadian Respiratory Journal* 8, 163–181.

Campbell, L. (1998) IV related phlebitis, complications and length of hospital stay: 2. *British Journal of Nursing* 7(22), 1364–1373.

Considine, J. (2005) The role of nurses in preventing adverse events related to respiratory dysfunction: Literature review, *Journal of Advanced Nursing* 49(6), 624–633.

Davies, A. (2009) How to manage patients with acute kidney injury. *Journal of Renal Nursing* 1(3), 119–122.

Dawson, J. and Christie, M. (2007) 'Just a sharp scratch': permanent radial, median and ulnar neuropathy following diagnostic venepuncture. *British Journal of Hospital Medicine* 68(3), 160–161.

Department of Health (2000) *Health Service Circular 2000/028: Resuscitation Policy*, 5 September. Department of Health, London.

Department of Health (2003a) *Winning Ways: Working Together To Reduce Healthcare Associated Infections In England*. Department of Health, London.

Clinical Skills for Nurses, First Edition. Claire Boyd

© 2013 John Wiley & Sons, Ltd. Published 2013 by John Wiley & Sons Ltd.

Department of Health (2005a) *Saving Lives: a Delivery Programme to reduce Healthcare Associated Infection including MRSA. High Impact Intervention Number 2b; Peripheral Line Care.* Department of Health, London.

Department of Health (2005b) *Saving Lives: Reducing Infection, Delivering Clean and Safe Care.* Department of Health, London.

Department of Health (2007) *Saving Lives: Reducing Infection, Delivering Clean and Safe Care. High Impact Intervention no. 5 urinary Catheter Care Bundle.* Department of Health, London.

Department of Health (2010a) *Six Years on: Delivering the Diabetes National Service Framework.* Department of Health, London.

Department of Health (2010) *The NHS Outcomes Framework 2011/12.* Department of Health, London.

Department of Health (2011) *Payment by Results Guidance for 2010/11.* Department of Health, London. www.dh.gov.uk/pbr.

Diabetes UK (2004) *Diabetes in the UK 2004: A Report from Diabetes UK, October 2004.* Diabetes UK, London.

Dougherty, L. (1996) Intravenous cannulation. *Nursing Standard* 11(20), 47–51.

Dougherty, L. (2011) Drug administration. In Dougherty, L. and Lister, S. (eds), *The Royal Marsden Hospital Manual of Clinical Nursing Procedures*, 8th edn. Wiley-Blackwell, Oxford.

Dougherty, L. and Lister, S. (eds) (2011) *The Royal Marsden Hospital Manual of Clinical Nursing Procedures*, 8th edn. Wiley-Blackwell, Oxford.

Dychter, S. et al. (2012) Intravenous therapy; a review of complications and economic considerations of peripheral access. *Journal of Infusion Nursing* 35(2), 84–91.

Eeles, R. (1994–present) *UK Generic Prostate Cancer Study.* Institute of Cancer Research and Royal Marsden NHS Foundation Trust, Surrey.

Glickman, S. and Kamm, M.A. (1996) Bowel dysfunction in spinal cord injury patients. *The Lancet* 347(9016), 1651–1653.

HMSO (2007) *Mental Capacity Act 2005 Code of Practice.* HMSO, London.

Home, P., Mant, J., Turner, C. et al. (2008) Management of Type 2 diabetes: summary of updated NICE guidelines. *British Medical Journal* 336, 1306–1308.

Ingram, P. and Lavery, I. (2005) Peripheral intravenous therapy: key risks and implications for practice. *Nursing Standard* 19(46), 55–64.

Institute for Healthcare Improvement (2011) *Early Warning Systems: Scorecards That Save Lives.* www.ihi.org/knowledge/Pages/ImprovementStories/EarlyWarningSystemsScorecardsThatSaveLives.aspx.

Mackay, C., Burke, D., Burke, J. et al. (2000) Association between the assessment of conscious level using the AVPU system and the Glasgow Coma Scale. *Pre-Hospital Immediate Care* 4, 17–19.

McCallum, L. and Higgins, D. (2012) Care of peripheral venous cannula sites. *Nursing Times* 108(34/35), 12–15.

Medicines and Healthcare Products Regulatory Agency (2005) *Report of the Independent Advisory Group on Blood Pressure Monitoring in Clinical Practice.* Department of Health, London.

Medicines and Healthcare Products Regulatory Agency (2007) *Intravascular and Epidural Devices Top Tips. Advice for Healthcare Professionals.* Department of Health, London.

Moore, T. (2003) Suctioning techniques for the removal of respiratory secretions. *Nursing Standard* 18(9), 47–53.

National Institute for Health and Clinical Excellence (2007a) *Faecal Incontinence: the Management of Faecal Incontinence in Adults.* NICE Clinical Guideline 49. NICE, London.

National Institute for Health and Clinical Excellence (2007b) *Acutely Ill Patients in Hospital: Clinical Guideline 50.* NICE, London.

National Institute for Health and Clinical Excellence (2010) *Lower Urinary Tract Symptoms: The Management of Lower Urinary Tract Symptoms in Men.* guidance.nice.org.uk/CG97.

National Patient Safety Agency (2007a) *Recognising and Responding Appropriately to Early Signs of Deterioration in Hospital Patients.* www.npsa.nhs.uk/EasySiteWeb/GatewayLink.aspx?alId=6240

National Patient Safety Agency (2007b) *Safer Care for the Acutely Ill Patient: Learning from Serious Incidents.* www.npsa.nhs.uk/EasySiteWeb/GatewayLink.aspx?alId=6241

National Patient Safety Agency (2009) *Female Urinary Catheters Causing Trauma to Adult Males.* Rapid Response Report NPSA/2009/RRR02. www.npsa.nhs.uk/nrls/alerts-and-directives/rapidrr/.

Nolan, J.P., Nadkarni, V.M., Billi, J.E. et al. (2010) International Consensus on Cardiopulmonary Resuscitation and Emergency Cardiovascular Care Science with Treatment Recommendations. Part 2; International Collaboration in Resuscitation Science. *Resuscitation* 81, 26–31.

Nursing and Midwifery Council (2002) *Guidelines for Records and Record Keeping.* NMC Publications, London.

Parker, G. (2008) An overview of female intermittent catheterisation. *Continence Essentials* 1, 60–65.

Peate, I. and Nair, M. (2011) *Fundamentals of Anatomy and Physiology for Student Nurses.* Wiley-Blackwell, Oxford.

Pellatt, G. (2007) Urinary elimination: part 2 – retention, incontinence and catheterisation. *British Journal of Nursing* 16(8), 480–485.

Preston, R. and Flynn, D. (2010) Observations in acute care: evidence based approach to patient safety. *British Journal of Nursing* 19(7), 442–447.

Royal College of Nursing (2003) *Standards for Infusion Therapy*. Royal College of Nursing, London.

Royal College of Nursing (2008a) *Bowel Care Including Digital Rectal Examination and Manual Evacuation of Faeces – Guidance for Nurses*. Royal College of Nursing, London.

Royal College of Nursing (2008b) *Catheter Care: RCN Guidance for Nurses*. Royal College of Nursing, London.

Royal College of Nursing (2010) *Standards for Infusion Therapy*. Tinyurl.com/RCN-infusion.

Scales, K. (2008) A practical guide to venepuncture and blood sampling. *Nursing Standard* 22(29), 29–36.

Serious Hazards of Transfusion. Annual reports 2010. Available at: www.shotuk.org.

Smith, J. and Roberts, R. (2011) *Vital Signs for Nurses – An Introduction to Clinical Observations*. Wiley-Blackwell, Oxford.

Spinal Cord Injury Centres of the United Kingdom and Ireland (2009) *Guidelines for Management of Neurogenic Bowel Dysfunction after Spinal Cord Injury*. Spinal Cord Injury Centres of the United Kingdom and Ireland.

St George's Healthcare NHS Trust (2006) *Guidelines for the Care of the Patient with Tracheostomy Tube. Portex*. St George's Healthcare NHS Trust, London.

Stainsby, D. et al. (2005) Reducing adverse events in blood transfusion. *British Journal of Haematology* 131, 8–12.

Tilley, S. and Watson, R. (2008) *Accountability in Nursing and Midwifery*, 2nd edn. Blackwell Science, Oxford.

Tortora, G.J. and Derrickson, B.H. (2010) *Essentials of Anatomy and Physiology*, 8th edn. John Wiley & Sons, New York.

Wiesel, P. and Bell, S. (2004) Bowel dysfunction: assessment and management in the neurological patient. In Norton, C. and Chelvanayagam, S. (eds), *Bowel Continence Nursing*. Beaconsfield Publishers, Beaconsfield.

WEBSITES

www.ALSG.org, Advanced Life Support Group

www.bcshguidelines.com, British Committee for Standards in Haematology Guidelines

www.bladderandbowelfoundation.org

www.mhra.gov.uk, Medicines and Healthcare Products Regulatory Agency

www.nice.org.uk, National Institute for Health and Clinical Excellence

www.npsa.nhs.uk, *Right Patient, Right Blood* evaluation reports

www.resus.org.uk, Resuscitation Council (UK)

Index

DEVELOPED BY STUDENTS FOR STUDENTS

You've made the right choice in selecting this Student Survival Skills book. Be sure to pick up the other books in the series to help you boost your competence both in the clinical skills lab and on your clinical placements – two core areas of your nursing education. The series is edited by Claire Boyd, a Practice Development Trainer in the Learning and Research Centre at North Bristol Healthcare Trust in the UK working closely with a team of practicing nurses and nursing students. Therefore, each handy pocket-sized book in the series includes words of wisdom and advice for real-life situations.

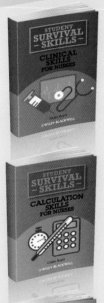

Clinical Skills for Nurses

Clinical Skills for Nurses covers the skills and procedures used most frequently in clinical practice, and includes Point of Care training; blood transfusion and tracheotomy care; venepuncture and peripheral cannulation; and early patient assessment and response. Each clear, concise chapter contains examples and questions based on what student nurses are likely to come across during clinical placements and in the clinical skills lab.

2013 • 9781118448779 • 224 pages

Calculation Skills for Nurses

Anxious about performing drug calculations? By clearly illustrating how mathematical theory relates to clinical nursing practice, *Calculation Skills for Nurses* enables you to calculate drug dosages with ease. Beginning with a review chapter for identification of key areas for further learning, each chapter takes the reader through a step-by-step journey of healthcare-related calculation exercises based on real-world situations.

2013 • 9781118448892 • 208 pages

Medicine Management Skills for Nurses

This essential guide explores the theory and practice of drug administration briefly and coherently, with 'test your knowledge' exercises and questions throughout to assess your learning. It also includes 'words of wisdom'- tips from real nursing students from their own experiences. Ideal for carrying to clinical placements and clinical areas, *Medicine Management Skills for Nurses* is your essential guide to the subject area of drugs and medicine administration.

2013 • 9781118448854 • 280 pages

Look out for **Communication Skills, Study Skills,** *and* **Care Skills** coming soon to the Student Survival Skills Series.

Digital editions are available for download to your computer or e-book reader. Please visit **www.wiley.com** or your preferred e-book vendor for further details or to purchase.

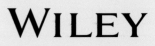

13-51286